Performing Arts Medicine in Clinical Practice

Howard A. Bird

Performing Arts Medicine in Clinical Practice

Springer

Howard A. Bird
University College London
London
UK

ISBN 978-3-319-12426-1 ISBN 978-3-319-12427-8 (eBook)
DOI 10.1007/978-3-319-12427-8

Library of Congress Control Number: 2015955266

Springer Cham Heidelberg New York Dordrecht London

Printed on acid-free paper

Springer International Publishing AG Switzerland is part of Springer Science+Business Media (www.springer.com)

Preface

Although written at the suggestion of the publisher, this book, which is designed to fill a specific need, is timely on several counts.
Performing Arts Medicine is a new but expanding speciality, which offers great challenges to the clinician and therapist in the service of the performer. It is closely related to Sports Medicine, and derives much from this discipline, established in the service of the athlete though perhaps also their financial sponsors. However, if the rules of the various sports are relatively rigid and the bodily requirements for the athletes and their injuries therefore broadly predictable, the art of the composer or choreographer is more flexible with fewer restrictions. Few would doubt that dancers were athletes. That professional musicians need to display equal athleticism, especially of the upper limb, is less generally recognized. This is before any consideration is given to the artistic temperament that often pushes the body to its limits.

The requirements for dance medicine differ somewhat from those for instrumental medicine (though not as much as might be thought) and the management of singers and even actors forms a third area of the speciality.

Practitioners inevitably come from many different backgrounds and are often performers themselves. Amongst the physicians, rheumatology and musculoskeletal medicine are important across all three areas, as is the need for help from orthopaedic surgeons. Singers and actors also fall into the province of the laryngologists. A sympathetic general practitioner is always invaluable. Physiotherapists, osteopaths and chiropracters all play an obvious important role though the importance of psychologists, dietitians and pharmacists is sometimes forgotten.

It is hoped this book will appeal to all of these disciplines, perhaps even providing simple didactic advice for others who feel insecure in this complicated niche area of medicine.

There has also been increasing interest in health from performers themselves. Dance Science, largely evolved from Sports Science, is now established at many Universities and Conservatoires in the United Kingdom. Musical Performance Science, much influenced by Dance Science, is still in its infancy but likely to expand quickly. All this has led to an increasing body awareness in the performers themselves, both in respect of anatomy and physiology, and it is hoped that they, as well as their teachers, will also find much in this book that is of interest.

A few enlightened organisations have attempted to nurture the speciality. In the United Kingdom, the efforts of the British Association for Performing Arts Medicine and Dance UK with their Healthier Dancer programme deserve particular mention. Although some medical schools have attempted to provide tuition, mainly through the components of the curriculum that the students select themselves, there is a need for broader post-graduate education in the field.

This has led to the recent establishment of an MSc degree in Performing Arts Medicine at University College, London, with the assistance of BAPAM and with the collaboration of the two partner institutions, the Royal College of Music and Trinity-Laban Conservatoire of Music and Dance. The author acts as a module leader on this degree course, and some of the contents of this book are derived from that syllabus.

The author, who has followed a career in Rheumatology at the University of Leeds, has had a life time interest in the medical problems of performers, and a recent Visiting Professorship at University College, London, in conjunction with their MSc course, has acted as a catalyst to write this book.

It does not aim to be a textbook or even fully comprehensive but explores areas of the speciality, mainly musculo-skeletal and sometimes controversial, that are of particular interest to the author and that illustrate principles in the management of this unique and sometimes demanding group of patient-performers. It attempts to provide a personal opinion alongside the established comprehensive textbooks. From the electronic version, individual chapters can be purchased separately so that those with interests only in one area of the speciality do not have to purchase the whole book.

The subject matter of the chapters is a personal selection and these are mixed with illustrative case histories, collected over some 30 years of clinical practice. It may not escape the attention of the reader that the author is also an amateur pianist.

I have tried to write in simple style so that all readers might find things of interest. The book is designed as a practical guide, without extensive references, though these are provided for some of the chapters. A reading list is also provided at the end for those wishing to take their knowledge to a more advanced level.

Any mistakes are entirely my own.

London, UK Howard A. Bird

Acknowledgements

Thanks are due:

To Suki Tyler, a clinical scientist and herself an ex-professional ballet dancer, for writing the majority of Chap. 3.

To Sofia Ornellas Pinto for help with Chap. 10.

To all patients who have offered themselves as case studies, or as clinical examples in the various chapters throughout this book, some of whom have also provided a commentary from the patient's viewpoint.

To Julia Megginson, Senior Editorial Assistant, and Melissa Morton, Commissioning Editor, and to all others who have helped at Springer, the publishers.

Finally, to my family for their tolerance.

Contents

Chapter 1
Expert Care of the Performing Artist

Although it is not always realised, the demands placed on the musculoskeletal system of performing artists at least resemble the demands placed upon elite athletes [1]. Moreover, the performer is driven according to the demands of the composer or choreographer, in turn interpreted by the conductor or artistic director to achieve a performance that delivers a profit for management. This contrasts with the world of sport where, to some extent, athletes can pace themselves in their training and events. Whilst dance requires athleticism of the whole body, musicians are largely athletes of the arms whilst singers and actors are athletes of the throat and larynx, though in some art forms such as physical theatre and circus, these boundaries are crossed. Arguably, the psychological demands on the performer are greater than those of the athlete, with stage fright always a potential concern.

Over recent decades sport has become increasingly commercialised. Top athletes now earn high salaries in many sports and, especially through sponsorship, professional baseball and football teams nowadays boast large financial turnovers. Increasingly, salaries in other sports tend not to lag behind. In turn, the peak health of the sportspeople has significant financial implications and, as a result, the speciality of sports medicine can attract high private income. Baseball teams and football teams retain an army of physicians,

H.A. Bird, *Performing Arts Medicine in Clinical Practice*,
DOI 10.1007/978-3-319-12427-8_1,

surgeons, psychologists and nutritionists who provide a worthwhile investment in the context of income that is accrued.

This is a far distance from the world of the performing artist. In the United Kingdom, only the largest ballet companies have finances to support a physiotherapist and smaller companies, particularly those for contemporary dance, will have no such facility, though may have insurance to cover the cost of urgent investigations required for acute injury in the hope that the 'show can go on'. For orchestras, AMABO (Association of Medical Advisers to British Orchestras), which is a voluntary organisation, nominates a general practitioner to work alongside each of the major symphony orchestras but otherwise care is rudimentary. Sports medicine has become a popular taught subject in medical schools; performing arts medicine remains neglected even though a previous background in arts subjects is no longer an impediment to recruitment to the profession. The care of musicians and dancers remains one of the greatest challenges in occupational musculoskeletal medicine.

Musicians at the highest level train frequently and compulsively. However, the diversity of instruments presents additional challenges, not least because although musicians come in different shapes and sizes instruments in general do not. Whilst nobody would deliberately purchase shoes that did not fit them, an instrumentalist may have to adapt to the size and weight of an instrument that does not suit them for long periods of playing. Some instruments also bring particular problems. Amongst woodwind instruments the flute, although light, is particularly difficult to hold, often requiring contorted positions of both arms for long periods. The left forearm is often hyperextended and the left wrist deviated radially, a recipe for compression neuropathy. Amongst the stringed instruments, the cello is amongst the most problematic, not least because of its awkward size, shape and need to be positioned between the legs, but also because the angle of playing required causes strain in the presence of any mild spinal scoliosis of the sort that afflicts many of the population. Brass players have problems with embouchure and thoracic excursion, although percussion normally provides a good job rotation apart from the use of the drum kit in popular music where the holding of the drum sticks often leads to overuse. Stringed instruments require asymmetric use of the arms, predisposing to quite different medical conditions on the left and right sides with the classical guitar particularly problematic in view of the wide finger stretches that are required of one hand [2–4].

In dance there is considerable variation between the different styles. Although many dancers receive a basic training either in ballet or contemporary dance, styles then divulge. The requirements for classical ballet differ considerably from those for modern ballet and within contemporary dance, the techniques required for Graham, Cunningham and Release are all different. Ethnic dance styles require further techniques and there is some overlap with martial arts and sports such as diving and gymnastics, which have an artistic component. In that the various options in these sports each attract a tariff, selection of a routine is to some extent in the hands of the performer who can choose a programme to best suit their musculoskeletal system, providing this commands sufficient potential marks to allow them to win the event [5–8].

The management of singers and even actors is a somewhat more specialised area. Clearly the skills of the ear, nose and throat specialist are crucial but attention to the musculoskeletal integrity of the chest which comprises the bellows is almost as important and often neglected. The larynx is essentially an articulation, its function in the elite performer controlled by striated muscle. This area also links closely with the embouchure problems that can be encountered by brass players.

The role of the composer or choreographer is clearly crucial and there is often an artistic incentive to push the body to the limits of its potential, even for the sake of spectacle. Where this collaboration is close, this may still be achieved in relative safety without any great risk of injury. One frequent problem in dance, however, is when a choreographer is employed to work with an original cast of a stage production, so the skills required are restricted to those of the performers. When a second cast, each of them of slightly different in body structure to the members of the original cast tasks over, unless funds allow for the choreography to be adjusted, injuries tend to occur. The piano works of composer/pianists who made a living by performing the music they composed (so invariably pushed their own technique to its limits) provide a insight into the wide inter-individual variation in the size, shape, and abilities of different hands.

Ethnicity attracts less attention but is equally important. There is a clear ethnic variation in joint laxity [9, 10] with those from the Indian sub-continent and African continent typically more lax than European Caucasians, though there is also ethnic variation in the sites of the body at which laxity is most pronounced. Laxity also seems to be pronounced in South-east Asiatic ethnic groups though this has been less well studied in the scientific literature even though it is well recognised in contemporary dance. Here the body build, strength and height all influence as well as the inter-racial variation in muscular structure, including a proportion of fast and slow twitch muscle fibres, which inform on both explosive power and endurance within dance.

It is perhaps not surprising that some sports and artistic activities reflect the specific ethnic characteristics of the participants. There is considerable variation in ethnic dance styles throughout the Far East as well as in the various martial arts that originated there. Capoeira, a combination of martial arts, dance and acrobatics, evolved as a method of restoring self-esteem in West African slaves in Brazil. There is a strong clinical impression that injuries are more frequent in Caucasians who attempt the sport than in those of West African or Brazilian extraction [11, 12].

In a move to train clinicians in this neglected yet complicated area of medicine, BAPAM (British Association for Performing Arts Medicine), a U.K. charity that has provided and subsidised clinics for performing artists for almost two decades, has combined with University College, London, to establish an MSc Course in Performing Arts Medicine. This is in close collaboration with the Royal College of Music and with Laban Conservatoire for Music and Dance where MSc degree courses in Science of Musical Performers and Dance Science already exist and more recently with Dance UK. These respective institutions [13, 14] cross fertilise modules and it is anticipated that ultimately, some teaching will be common for each of these separate courses. Details of the course are available on the website of University College, London at www.ucl.ac.uk/surgicalscience/departments_research/iseh/msc_performing_arts_medicine.

The degree of MSc in Performing Arts Medicine is currently offered as a full-time course for 1 year or a part-time course for 2 years. It includes modules in anatomy, physiology, psychology, therapy and drug treatment and one-third of the time is spent in original research. There is an opportunity to attend specialised clinics for voice, dance and musicians and students have the option of specialising in one of these three areas if they choose to. The course, which is currently in its second year, has so far attracted doctors, physiotherapists, chiropractors and osteopaths as well as an Alexander Technique teacher. Many of these students are also performers at a near professional standard. In view of the specialised nature of the course, applications are also considered from those with a wide range of first degrees as well as from those with a masters degree in either Dance Science or Music Science even if they have no medical qualifications. Recently at least half of the students have been from abroad, many from Europe but some from further afield.

One-third of the time is spent in research and this is already producing original research in many new areas, intriguingly often in areas of performance at which the students themselves excel, providing particular added value when the research is conducted in an area where the student already has substantial expertise.

A large part of this book is based upon lectures given as part of one of the modules of this course. It is to be hoped that ultimately these individuals might go on to become the professors and consultants in Performing Arts Medicine of the future.

A question sometimes raised is whether such specialist training is absolutely necessary. Clearly some training is desirable and any is better than none but with many practitioners ill at ease when confronted with even an amateur performer. Time and a sympathetic ear are always appreciated by performers who invariably have a close understanding of their own body and its capabilities. However, a clinician who is also a performer, in whatever genre, is more likely to have an instinctive understanding of the psychological needs of performers and the pressures under which they have to work. They may also be in a position to review the musical score or the choreography to determine the cause of any injury. Moreover if the clinician has a sufficiently high standard of technique, they can to a certain extent double as therapist and technique teacher. Otherwise one way forward may be the development of specialist clinics where a clinician joins a technique teacher in a clinic themed to a particular instrument or group of instruments or to a particular style of dance.

References

1. Bird HA. Editorial: the performing artist as an elite athlete. Rheumatology. 2009;48:1469–70.
2. Tubiana R, Amadio PC, editors. Medical problems of the instrumental musician. London: Martin Dunitz Ltd; 2000 (626 pages).
3. Greer JM, Panush RS. Musculoskeletal problems of performing artists. Baillieres Clin Rheumatol. 1994;8:103–35.
4. Winspur I, Wynn Parry CB. The musician's hand: a clinical guide. London: Martin Dunitz Ltd; 1998 (201 pages).
5. Washington EL. Musculoskeletal injuries in theatrical dancers: site, frequency, and severity. Am J Sports Med. 1978;6:75–98.
6. Bowling A. Injuries to dancers: prevalence, treatment, and perceptions of causes. Br Med J. 1989;298:731–4.
7. Steele VA. Injury amongst female Olympic style competitive gymnasts. MSc thesis, Physical Education Section/University of Salford; 1984.
8. Howse J. Dance technique and injury prevention. 3rd ed. London: A & C Black; 2000 (212 pages).

9. Schweitzer G. Laxity of metacarpophalangeal joints of fingers and interphalangeal joint of the thumb: a comparative inter-racial study. S Afr Med J. 1970;44:246–9.
10. Wordsworth P, Ogilvie D, Smith R, Sykes B. Joint mobility with particular reference to racial variation and inherited connective tissue disorders. Br J Rheumatol. 1987;26:9–12.
11. Bird HA, Walker A, Newton J. A controlled study of joint laxity and injury in gymnasts. J Orthop Rheumatol. 1988;1:139–45.
12. Bird HA. Hypermobility in the performing arts and sport. In: Beighton P, Grahame R, Bird H, editors. Hypermobility of joints. 3rd ed. London: Springer; 1999. p. 125–45.
13. Williamon A. Musical excellence: strategies and techniques to enhance performance. Oxford: Oxford University Press; 2004. p. 1–299.
14. Watson AHD. The biology of musical performance and performance-related injury. Lanham: Scarecrow Press Inc; 2009 (367 pages).

Chapter 2
Musical Instruments and Their Demands on the Body

Introduction

On the basis that the practitioner needs at least some understanding of the artistic demands placed on the performer, the next three chapters briefly discuss potential strains placed on the body by instruments, dance and singing respectively. This informs on the stresses of the art form and often, therefore, the propensity for injury.

Some basic principles apply. In the case of musical instruments a major problem is that in general musical instruments come in standard shapes and sizes whilst performers differ in size and body build. It follows that the biomechanical strain exerted by each instrument will vary from player to player. In turn, constitutionally, certain players may be better suited to playing some instruments rather than others. This, a basic principle in selection for elite sport, has so far largely eluded the musical profession. By the time music students reach a conservatoire, it is usually too late to change to an instrument that might suit their body better.

It is unusual not to be able to find a technical cause for an injury or strain even if the diagnosis is only "overuse syndrome", discussed in more detail in Chap. 6. One common cause is interchange between two instruments requiring similar technique for playing but differing slightly in size and weight. Examples are interchange between the violin and the

H.A. Bird, *Performing Arts Medicine in Clinical Practice*,
DOI 10.1007/978-3-319-12427-8_2,

viola, the oboe and the cor anglais and the clarinet and the saxophone. This last is not just a matter of size and weight. The clarinet is played in a relatively erect physiological position; the saxophone is heavier and also requires a slight spinal rotation, unsuited to minor degrees of natural spinal twist.

This all comes before consideration of the more familiar contributors to injury such as tiredness, stress, trans-meridional travel without acclimatization and inadequate preparation without warm-up.

Consideration of the demands of the actual music being played is also important, hence the desirability of matching the symptoms with the musical score. An instrument such as the piano has not only evolved over the years, but the demands made by composers have also become more complex. Often just a small section of music lasting only a few bars, or a particular movement of a sonata can be the single crucial factor in producing overuse or injury during a much longer recital.

Most performers, invariably intelligent and with good body awareness, understand this. Beware the doctor who fails to listen to the performers analysis of the problem! Even if this is not described in precise medical terms, it invariably provides a clue and ultimately the performers analysis is usually correct in view of their intuitive understanding of technique.

Stringed Instruments

Unusually amongst the different groups of instruments, stringed instruments require quite different functions from the two arms. This is analogous to the problems encountered in sports medicine with racquet sports. Most other instruments require symmetrical playing. Problems at the left shoulder and right forearm in a violinist are unlikely to have resulted from the instrument. Problems at the right shoulder (the bowing arm) and left forearm may well have done.

The Violin and Viola

The difference in size and weight between these two instruments has already been mentioned as a risk factor for those who mainly play one but occasionally the other. Problems tend to occur at the right shoulder, though shoulder function should always be considered in relation to the whole shoulder girdle as well as the upper thoracic and cervical spine. In the left arm problems mainly occur with the forearm muscles and their tendons. Although data from music clinics sometimes suggests disproportionate numbers of injuries in violinists, this is probably more a reflection of the large number of musicians who play the violin. A variety of chin rests are available which often relieve musculo-skeletal symptoms in the spine, shoulders and even arms.

The Cello

Arguably this is the most problematic of the stringed instruments. The pattern of injuries resembles those from the violin, often compounded by the greater forces required by the heavier and longer strings. But a greater problem is that the instrument, which needs to be played with a slight rotation of the spine, anchors the pelvis which in turn limits the flexibility required in the lower spine. Cellists who have a slight natural rotation of the spine in the wrong direction seem to be especially at risk of mechanical overuse and therefore low back pain.

The Double Bass

By contrast double bass players are relatively injury free. The instrument is played at an angle and the strings are the heaviest of all. But unlike the cello which fixes the body, the bass player is able to adjust the angle of the spine by rotating slightly on their stool. The jazz bass player, who usually stands, has additional movement options available to him to reduce the strain of playing in a fixed awkward position.

Guitars

The classical guitar, mainly requiring use of the hands and fingers, emphasizes the asymmetry of the two sides to a high degree. The main problem is the lateral laxity required of the stretched fingers in the left hand, still needing to exert some considerable force on the metal strings. Those with hypermobile hands, often selected because of their prowess with this instrument, seem to be at particular risk of overuse syndromes. For popular music, a wide variety of other guitars exist, some much heavier and larger than the classical guitar. Although similar problems occur with them, these often seem to be less severe, perhaps because the technique required is less exacting.

The Harp

Although only occasionally encountered, this instrument causes a unique set of problems. It is a large instrument played a little from the side, with the slightly twisted spine relatively fixed. The plucking of the strings requires that the thumbs are often slightly hyperextended whilst exerting considerable force so thumb base problems are common. Finally the need for the feet to reach and operate the several fixed pedals (Fig. 2.1) puts further strain on the position of the spine and the legs.

Woodwind Instruments

This group of instruments are broadly symmetrical and all require considerable dexterity of both hands. Moreover, a reliable supply of wind is required so the lungs, chest and diaphragm which together provide the bellows, also need to

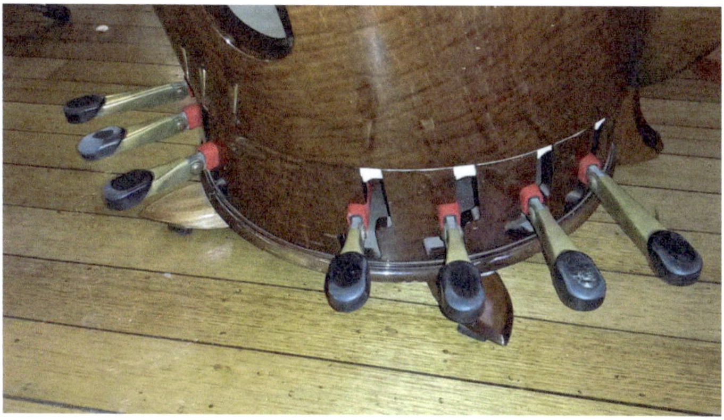

FIGURE 2.1 The pedals on the harp

be functional. Good lip control is required to produce the tone.

The Piccolo

The smallest and lightest member of the family, this is held at a most awkward angle but most players seem to adapt because it is so short. Small hands are an advantage and the reason so few injuries are seen probably reflects the limited use of it made by composers in orchestral scores.

The Flute

The most problematic instrument of the group, this is also held in a most awkward position but is sufficiently long to act as a brace between the hands and the mouth. Only when the player has arms of exactly appropriate length is it problem free. Most players need to contort the elbows and wrists into un-anatomical positions for the long periods that the instrument is required in most orchestral scores. A variety of aids and adaptions are available and are often used by flautists (Fig. 2.2).

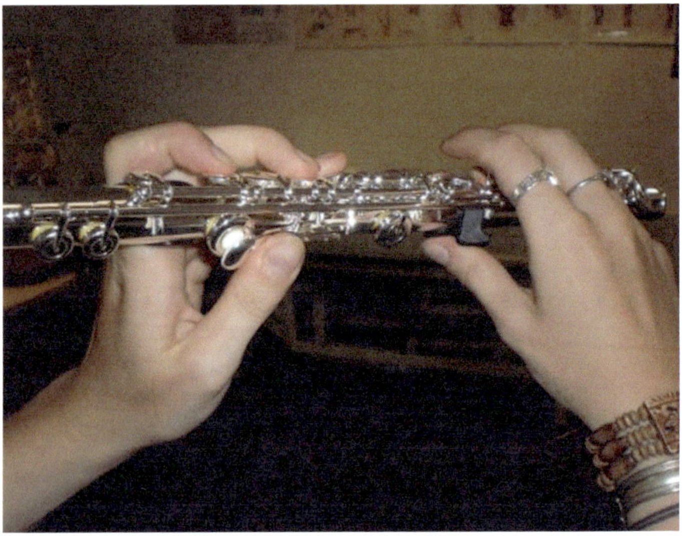

FIGURE 2.2 Playing the flute with adaptions

The Oboe and Cor Anglais

By contrast to the lighter woodwind instruments, both are held in an easy functional position, the cor anglais heavier and a little more awkward. Few injuries seem to occur. The double reed is much less supported at the lips than the single reed of the clarinet so overuse problems of the lips are common. It is sometimes forgotten that this is a nine-fingered instrument. The weight of the instrument is mainly supported by the static right thumb.

The Clarinet

The instrument is held in an easy functional position so few injuries occur and the lips (and single reed) are rested against the instrument, reducing strain on the lips. Like the elbow the right thumb is static and supports the weight of the instrument. Most hands are of a size to adapt to the various holes and levers; strain is most often encountered with those fingers operating the longest keys in players with small hands.

The Saxophone Family

The prototype and most familiar instrument, the "alto sax" is essentially a metal clarinet, though it is heavier and played at a slight angle against the spine. This can cause problems in clarinet players with mild spinal twist or deformities. It is not always realized that there is a large family of saxophones, some comparable in size to a small clarinet, others comparable to the larger brass instruments.

The Bassoon

This double reed instrument is more likely to cause embouchure problems, both because of the relatively unsupported reed and the size of the instrument. It causes relatively few musculo-skeletal problems, perhaps because, like the double bass, musicians can adjust their spine around the instrument

Brass Instruments

A heavier group of instruments compared to their respective woodwind counterparts of similar pitch so breath production and control become even more important. The strain on the lips required to produce the sound in these metal instruments is considerable so brass players can have major problems with embouchure, which impinges on the expertise of the ear nose and throat specialist. They also require specific techniques of the tongue. The group of instruments is asymmetric in terms of musculo-skeletal function, one hand usually operating the valves while the other is static or supporting the instrument. The trombone requires considerable versatility of one shoulder.

The French Horn

The right hand stops the bell while the left operates the valves. Much of the sound derives from the lips and the instrument is notoriously unreliable compared to all others, the orchestral writing often exposed and of long duration. Arguably, this is the instrument that might most easily predispose to stage fright.

The Cornet and Trumpet

The right hand operates the valves and the left hand supports in both instruments. As with most groups of brass instruments there are many variations in size and weight. Musculoskeletal problems in the arms are minimal and mainly associated with the production and control of the breath as well as the embouchure.

The Trombone

Potentially the most problematic instrument for the joints because the right shoulder controls the pitch by adjusting the length of the metal tube so needs both strength and flexibility, not needed in the other shoulder which mainly just stabilises the instrument.

The Tuba

The right hand operates the valves and the left arm supports the weight of this and similar large brass instruments. Breath control and embouchure are both crucial.

Keyboards

These are symmetric instruments requiring dexterity of the fingers and in the case of the organ pedals movement of the legs from the hips down. The piano is essentially a percussive instrument though capable of much variation in tone.

The Piano

Factors that contribute to injury are the action (the force required to depress a note), the regulation (this force should be equal for all notes on the keyboard), and the height and the position of the piano stool. The smaller piano often requires a greater percussive force; the largest concert grand pianos require little force to play as they have such massive resonating sounding boards. Injuries can occur as high as the shoulder, but usually involve the forearms and the fingers with their tendon apparatus. Overuse is usually symmetric, affecting both arms. Any spinal twist may require a change from the normal piano stool to a duetting stool, which allows the pelvis to slide from side to side (Fig. 2.3) or to a stool that rotates which is of especial value for a corkscrew twist in the spine (Fig. 2.4). An electronic keyboard rarely has the same type of action as a piano with conventional hammers and springs and a change from one to the other can predispose to overuse injuries.

The Organ

The use of the foot pedals can lead to problems in the legs. Usually, however, problems are restricted to the forearms since the instrument is not so percussive as the piano. Indeed, because there is no facility for continued resonance when a key is released, the style of playing is quite different with more smoothness of finger movement to achieve a legato

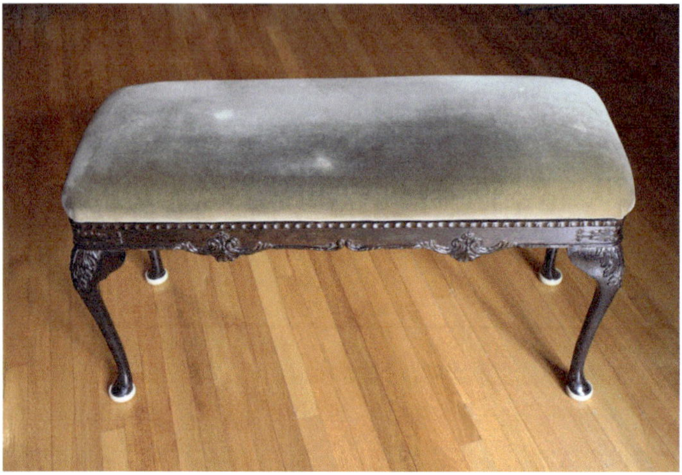

FIGURE 2.3 A piano stool that allows the pianist to slide

effect. Lateral movement of each finger assumes more importance.

Percussion

Orchestral percussionists tend to be required sparingly by composers. So there is time to recuperate and with the exception of drummers, percussionists are only occasionally seen in Performing Arts clinics.

Tympani

The drums are struck from a position of mechanical advantage and are arranged around the performer so there are no great risks.

Struck Percussion

This tends to be a perfect job rotation with only sort bursts of activity, hence no great risk factors for repetitive strains.

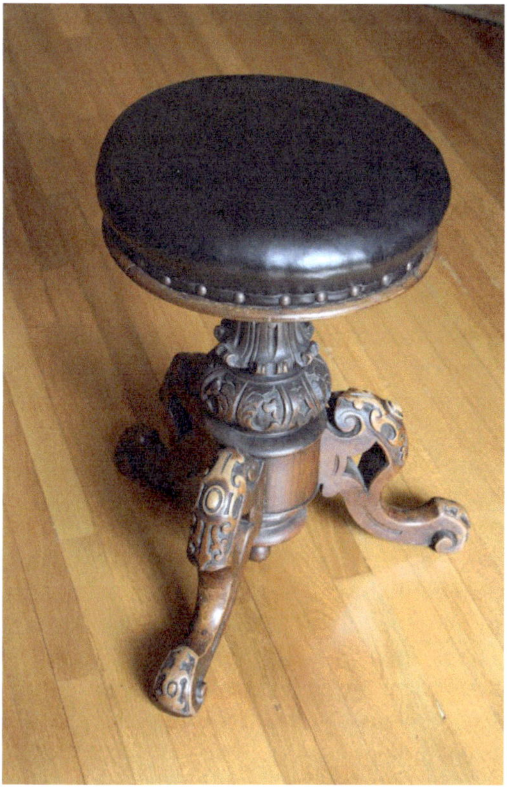

FIGURE 2.4 A piano stool that allows the pianist to rotate

Tuned Percussion

Comprising the xylophone, glockenspiel and marimba, this has elements of keyboard practice which can be quite demanding in terms of technique. The holding of the hammers can be a particular problem.

Drum Kit

This is almost the only instrument that can be arranged around the performer and adjusted for the height and body shape. However, in popular music it is the backbone of the performance and extremely repetitive. The main problem is the holding of the sticks. Although there are several different grips that can be tried, drum kit players are susceptible to a variety of hand problems associated with grip. A change to a different technique or adaptions to the drumsticks may assist.

Coda

This survey has mainly considered the instruments most commonly encountered in Performing Arts clinics. Space has not allowed consideration of some families of instruments, for example the recorder family, and it will be apparent that there are many variations on each of the common instruments, not always required in orchestral scores, though perhaps allowing some variation in solo work.

Nevertheless, many injuries encountered in clinics devoted to musicians could be categorized as "overuse injuries" (considered in more detail in Chap. 6), not least because professional players spend long hours devoted to practice, then rehearsal and then performance. It remains a strong impression that only a small proportion of performers are exactly suited to the ergonomics of their chosen instrument, that choice of instrument often made for a variety of reasons, none likely to involve detailed consideration of ergonomics. It even remains a theoretical possibility that in children the choice of instrument should involve consideration of the child's anatomy and physiology as would be expected in the selection for elite training squads in sport.

This is perhaps a more realistic strategy for preventing injury in later professional life than the fanciful redesigning of instruments on ergonomic grounds though a variety of simple devices are available to assist performers, some of which will be considered in Chap. 5.

Chapter 3
Styles of Dance and Their Demands on the Body

Introduction

Dance has evolved in many different forms, with wide variations in technique, style and artistic expression. These differences are what distinguish the dance type, its cultural origins and artistic purpose: a ballet dancer's use of pointe work and extension creates a sense of etherealism on stage, while an Afro-Caribbean dancer's low centre of gravity and rhythmic foot stamping highlights the connection with the earth and story telling. Because of these individual, highly stylized techniques, there are very specific physical demands placed on the body. Flexibility, strength and power, cardiovascular fitness, body composition, ethnicity and aesthetics are all factors that contribute to different dance styles in varying degrees. Some dancing communities may be more exacting in their requirements with regards to length and intensity of training, age and physical characteristics or emotional maturity and musicality. For example, ballet requires high levels of external rotation in the hip, both for aesthetic and functional purposes. Poorly developed 'turn-out' is a leading cause of injury in ballet so strength must be developed over years of training to prevent compensatory overload on the knees and ankles. Contemporary dance utilizes the floor a great deal as a choreographic tool, requiring the dancer to fall and roll,

Written in collaboration with Suki Tyler

H.A. Bird, *Performing Arts Medicine in Clinical Practice*,
DOI 10.1007/978-3-319-12427-8_3,

often with unpredictable changes in speed and direction. Core stability, flexibility and strength in the legs and ankles are of paramount importance to perform these movements well, and to protect the knees as much as possible.

Apart from the technical demands of dance, other factors such as costume requirements, performance conditions such as the rake of the stage and the psychological stress of a dancer's lifestyle can all take their toll on the body. Healthcare professionals, including doctors, who treat this unique sub-set of performing artists should be fully aware of the specific demands associated with each dance form in order to make a comprehensive diagnosis.

A full discussion of the medical aspects of every type of dance is beyond the scope of this short chapter. It will therefore consider ballet in some depth, before moving to modern dance, mainly contemporary. The aim is to provide an insight into the technique required by dancers and their problems in a style to which the principles of medical care can then be applied.

Ballet: Athletic and Aesthetic

Ballet is arguably one of the most exacting forms of dance in terms of body type, aesthetic detail and length of training required to perform professionally. Ever increasing demands for technical virtuosity and anatomical beauty are creating a generation of highly competitive and incredibly athletic ballet dancers. Well arched feet, high leg extensions, multiple pirouettes and feather-like jumps are all hallmarks of ballet and its quest for perfection. However, with this pursuit of 'effortless' beauty on stage comes strain on the body, both physiologically and psychologically. Repetitive back bends and gravity-defying arabesques can plave serious strain on the lumbar spine, potentially leading to joint or ligament damage. Constant 'turn-out' of the hips can strain ligaments of the supporting knees, feet and ankles. And an emphasis on low body weight, particularly for female dancers, may adversely affect hormonal balance and increase risk of fractures. These are just some examples of the demands of classical ballet technique and their possible deleterious effects upon the body. We will now discuss ballet technique in more depth, its training methods, performance factors and the ramifications for the professional dancer.

Technique

The classical ballet style is instantly recognizable by its grace, elegance and symmetrical line of the body. It's characterized by three fundamental elements: the lengthened spine and high centre of gravity; externally rotated hips ('turn-out'); and the maximally plantar-flexed foot ('pointe').

Whatever height the dancer may be, 'lifting' and 'lengthening' through the spine is one of the foundations of classical technique, allowing mobility of movement and creating that effortless, ethereal quality of ballet. A high centre of gravity and lengthened back muscles help to reduce the curves of the spine, and thus their vulnerability to injury when forces are applied, as in jumps, twists, extensions and pirouettes. It also sets up the correct weight distribution, slightly forward on the toes, and engagement of the correct supporting or working muscles. Additionally, it helps to provide momentum for turns and jumps. The resulting lightness of movement, characterized by both male and female ballet dancers, is a quality that not only masks the effort going into the performance, but actually reduces the effort itself, preventing potential injury. A dancer who 'sinks' into their hips in pirouettes or lands heavily in jumps is not going to get through a three act ballet intact. Muscles will be working inefficiently, joints will be strained and the dancer will be utterly exhausted. Young dancers must master this correct posture from the very beginning of their training, ensuring proper spinal alignment and weight distribution. If this is not achieved then not only will the dancer struggle with more complex technique, but the forces of movement will be ineffectively transmitted through the joints, incorrect muscles will be engaged, predisposing to injury, particularly of the back and lower limbs.

External rotation of the hips, or turn-out, is another foundation of ballet technique – without it, the art form would not be recognizable. It originates from King Louis XIV's 'Sun King' performance, where he adopted the style of outwardly pointed feet to show off his shoe buckles. All classical positions require it for aesthetic purposes – to display the beauty of the feet and legs – as well as functionally allowing greater range of movement, stabilization of the lower limb and engagement of specific target muscles. The shape of the ball-and-socket joint of the hip, the elasticity of the surrounding joint capsule and ligaments and the strength of the internal and external rotator muscles all affect the possible range of turnout in a dancer. Ideally they will have a minimum of 60° external rotation of the hip in order to pursue a career in classical ballet. If there is a limited amount of available turn-out, or if the turn-out is not supported correctly by the internal and external hip rotators, the likelihood of injury to the spinal column, knees, ankles and feet becomes very high.

One of the most distinguishing features of classical ballet is the plantar-flexed (pointed) foot. The dancer's feet are highly articulated and they use them as sensitively as the hand to rebound, absorb shock and support the body. In order to do this, they exercise the feet through full dorsiflexion to plantar-flexion, thousands of times throughout the day. A highly arched instep and flexible ankle produce a beautiful line of the leg, visually extending the leg muscles and contributing to the ethereal image of the 'floating' dancer. Females go all the way up onto 'pointe', at maximum plantar-flexion, supported by pointe shoes. To accomplish this takes many years of training, stretching and strengthening all the intrinsic muscles of the feet, as well those of the ankles, legs and core. Despite the highly mobile foot being favoured aesthetically in ballet, it brings with it a lot of inherent instability. Young dancers attempting pointe work too early, when their strength has not been sufficiently developed, may cause undue strain on their joints, ligaments and muscles, and ankle injuries are the most common of all injuries in ballet.

Dancers, like athletes, require immense amounts of cardiovascular fitness, strength, power, speed and flexibility to perform the well-known classics like Swan Lake, Nutcracker and The Sleeping Beauty. The ballet movements themselves can range from the slow ('adagio') and controlled, such as languorous extensions, expressive arms and back ('port-de-bras') and enduring balances, to the fast paced and dexterous, including jumping, turning and intricate footwork. Both require muscular endurance as well as speed and power, coupled with substantial flexibility. Typically, the intermittent, high intensity nature of dancing in a full length ballet will utilize both the aerobic and anaerobic systems. Corps-de-ballet members, the 'body' of the ballet, are most often required to perform in unison, mirroring each other exactly, whether it be in fast-paced, high energy enchainements or when standing motionless in line while the soloists perform. This requires both endurance and power, and of course immense concentration. In Act II of Swan Lake for example, it is possible for muscles to seize up and body temperature to cool when holding the standing positions for a long period of time when an immediate change of pace requiring explosive power and flexibility could potentially result in injury. Soloists and principals may get more recovery time in the wings between their solos and pas-de-deux, but this is not always the case. A ballet like Kenneth MacMillan's 'Manon' requires the lead female role to perform almost throughout the entire performance.

The style of choreography in different ballets can vary immensely. Some require very 'classical' placement in terms of lines of the body, height of extensions, use of the upper body and hip positioning; others push the boundaries of the classical technique, encouraging more freedom of movement and expression, daring the dancer to use their bodies in completely new ways. There may also be particular artistic demands from the choreographer, in terms of musicality and quality of movement. For example, Frederick Ashton's 'La

Fille Mal Gardee' displays the English classical style at its best, with emphasis on clean lines, articulated upper body movements, intricate footwork and a very lyrical, controlled quality. This technical precision is difficult to achieve, and will easily highlight any flaws in a dancer's technique. Nimble feet are essential, and a lack of strength may predispose to lower limb injury. In contrast, Balanchine's 'Jewels' is much more fast-paced, showing off the dramatic athleticism of the dancer, the high, open extensions in arabesque and hypermobile back and arms. Joint range of motion is pushed to the limit, jumps are high and powerful rather than delicate and ethereal, and spins are executed with much more momentum. The dancer's body is taking a huge amount of force from all angles, and injuries may spread to the hips, back and shoulders.

The roles and technical requirements of the male and female dancer typically differ in ballet, and consequently gender-specific injuries are common. Traditionally the female must dance on pointe, and there is a greater emphasis on higher extensions and the beautiful, 'feminine' lines of the legs, feet and upper back. Strain on the hips, knees and ankles are therefore much more prevalent, particularly those with hypermobility and joint laxity. The male on the other hand does not have to display such flexibility, but as the 'danseur noble' he shows his strength and power through much higher jumps and multiple turns. In addition, he must partner the female in 'pas-de-deux' work, supporting and often lifting her above head height. All of this can put a great deal of pressure on the lower back, so extra weight training in the gym is a necessary component of a male dancer's core training.

Training

A ballet dancer should start training well before the age of 10, and ideally full-time from the age of 11, in order to gain the necessary strength, flexibility and artistic maturity required of the art form. As discussed before, ballet is very exacting in its standards, and in this pursuit of perfection, certain physical characteristics, as well as musicality and a love for dance are a prerequisite. Ballet schools will scrupulously assess young dancers during auditions, favouring those with a high level of natural turn out and flexibility, high arches of the feet, long legs with a relatively short torso, long neck, and a general slim physique. In the past, ballet was dominated by dancers of Caucasian origin, most likely due to its European roots and elitist ideals. It was thought that dancers from other parts of the world perhaps did not have the required physiques demanded of ballet, nor the correct 'look' on stage. Thankfully, times have changed, and more and more dancers from African, Asian, central and southern American origin are performing in the world's top ballet companies.

Because of these aesthetic pressures to maintain a slim physique, particularly for female ballet dancers who need to be lifted by their partners, there is a risk of sub-optimal nutrition and potentially disordered eating. Low body weight combined with high levels of athletic activity can result in certain medical conditions such as amenorrhea, osteoporosis and higher risk of stress fractures. Childhood and adolescence are periods of opportunity and vulnerability for establishing bone health, so the trainee dancer needs particular support then. Rigorous training schedules, inadequate nutrition and repetitive loading of developing bones may cause fractures, most commonly in the metatarsals and tibia. Fractures of the base of the second metatarsal may occur more frequently in younger dancers who start pointe work too early. It is imperative that low body weight and menstrual irregularities are addressed through adequate nutritional advice with support from teachers.

A dancer's training consists predominantly of daily class, where they learn the ballet technique. It includes a series of set exercises of increasing intensity and difficulty, at the barre then into the centre, choreographed slightly differently by each teacher. The format has hardly changed over several hundred years, with a strong emphasis on discipline, structure, repetition and formality. The teacher sets the exercise, the dancers perform and then the teacher critiques. Some teachers are stricter than others, preferring to emphasise flaws rather than offer praise, as a means to getting the best out of the dancer. To the younger, more vulnerable ballerina, this psychology may be hard to deal with, potentially leading to issues of low self-esteem and depression. As the dancer matures, they must learn how to deal with the negativity and disappointment that are intrinsic to the subjective world of ballet; not all directors or choreographers will like them, whether it's because of technique, their 'look' or even their personality. Resilience is key to the longevity of a dancer's career.

Other Factors

Ballet was first performed in the French courts during the seventeenth century. It then later moved to theatres, with flat or raked stages surrounded by a vast auditorium. Learning to deal with all the challenges of stage performances is just part of the dancer's daily life. Often the young dancer will get their first experiences of performance on stage while at ballet school, and it can be quite a shock! After years of practising in mirrored studios, in simple leotards and tights, surrounded just by their teacher and contemporaries, the theatre can be a nerve-racking ordeal. Even for the seasoned professional dancer, adjusting to the stage can sometimes be a demanding process.

Choreography must first be marked on stage, as the space available may be quite different to that of the studio. Jumps and turns may have to 'travel' more or less; movement arcs may be shallower or deeper; scenery and props must be navigated. Without this adjustment process, a dancer may be at real risk of being injured or causing injury to other dancers. Particularly in pas-de-deux, distance and timing is imperative, and any discrepancy between either partner may be disastrous. Throw a raked stage into the mix and the propensity for injury is compounded as the dancer's centre of balance is challenged. Minute adjustments in turns, balances and jump landings must be made as a result of the unfamiliar gravitational pulls, and travelling upstage becomes a lot harder work. More than anything though, the raked stage may present a real psychological problem to the dancer – and fear of their upcoming performance could negatively affect their technique and cause injury.

Lighting can be another challenge. A pitch black auditorium combined with blinding spotlights on stage can easily throw a dancer's sense of balance. Spotting in turns is imperative to reduce dizziness, and locating a good 'spot' can often be difficult in a sea of darkness – the theatre 'exit' signs are usually the only option. The famous 32 fouettes performed by Odile in Swan Lake are challenging enough in the studio, but when combined with all of these factors on stage, are really quite an impressive feat! The heat intensity of the lights can also exacerbate performance related dehydration, and adequate water intake is very important.

Ballet costumes are all part of the artistic creation on stage. Since the birth of ballet, costumes have changed dramatically, with increasing emphasis on revealing the dancer's form and beauty of line. As such, the costumes these days are made to be as streamlined as possible, allowing maximum freedom of movement. If they are not fitted correctly, this may impede a dancer's technique and predispose to injury. In the classical ballets, females will often be in some form of tutu, depending on the style. In Giselle, for example, the skirt is longer and fuller, portraying a more romantic image, while in Swan Lake the tutu is more pancake shaped, displaying the full leg and the virtuosity of the dancer. Men will most likely be in tights and some form of jacket. The character dancers will often be in more elaborate clothing; these costumes may be much heavier, headdresses more substantial. A corps-de-ballet member may be a peasant in Act I of Swan Lake, wearing a weighty character skirt and heeled character shoes, followed by a quick change into a tutu and pointe shoes for a swan in Act II, and then back into character for Act III's palace ball. The style and feel of movement in these three costumes will be quite different, placing different demands on the body. The feet may swell slightly in character shoes, making it harder for the dancer to fit them back into pointe shoes and articulate the feet as required in Act II. Also, costumes can cause some issues in pas-de-deux work – the male dancer may often get a face-full of tulle when lifting his partner above his head, impairing his vision and sense of balance. If his own costume is slightly restrictive in the shoulders, he may struggle to lift effectively, placing extra strain upon his lower back and making it unsafe for the female.

Another important aspect of performance is the psychological impact on a dancer. Commonly, ballet dancers are highly sensitive perfectionists and mentally, this can often lead to a generalized anxious state if not adequately controlled. Stress caused by body image, workload, fear of failure or fear of injury can easily build up in the dancer's mind. And when this is combined with fear of an audience on stage, performance anxiety can seriously affect their technique. Muscles may tense and seize up, breathing may become laboured and the dancer will struggle to produce efficient movement. Positive mental imagery, breathing techniques, relaxation and support from others may all go some way to reducing anxiety in a dancer.

A professional ballet career will also most likely include touring and performing in different theatres and in different countries. Some companies will tour extensively, transporting their dancers, costumes and sets all around the world. Others may tour less frequently, especially if they have their own 'home' theatre. Often the more famous principal dancers will be asked to guest perform with other companies. Consequently, the ballet dancer must be adaptable to ever changing living, rehearsal and performance conditions.

One of the main challenges of touring is the risk of fatigue. Extensive travelling, especially across time zones, can really affect a dancer's sleep patterns, and thus their physical and mental acuity. Additionally, rest and recovery are essential elements in a dancer's daily life, and if these are cut short by intermittent performance schedules, then they are at real risk of exhaustion and sub-optimal dancing. Finding accommodation may be an added stress and living conditions may not be ideal, with dancers often sharing rooms because of financial pressure. With such a change in routine, dancers may struggle to 'switch off' or at least get some proper down-time alone to recuperate.

New environments with different cultures and languages may also cause problems, especially when it comes to buying food and other essentials. Dancers, like athletes, have a finely tuned diet that provides all the energy and nutrients they need to perform and maintain their physiques. Certain foods may become more difficult to obtain and any new flavours and ingredients may seem strange to the palate, discouraging eating. Low energy, lack of nutrients and potential stomach upsets all pose a risk to a dancer's performance. Their immune function may become impaired, increasing their susceptibility to poor health and injury.

The weather may be an important factor too. Touring to colder countries, such as Scandinavia, can create problems. Extra warm-up preparation may be required before class and performance to ensure muscles have not seized up outside in the cold conditions. More protective clothing must be worn inside the studio and out, alongside adequate footwear to prevent the risk of slipping on snow and ice and causing injury. In contrast, hot or tropical weather may cause dancers to become dehydrated and lethargic, so replacing water and electrolytes becomes essential. If studios are not well ventilated, sweat may accumulate on the floor and make it treacherous, especially during large jumping and turning sequences. A three act ballet may become even more of a marathon than it normally is. Heavy costumes will become drenched in sweat and even pointe shoes may disintegrate at a faster pace, so dancers really need time to acclimatize to the conditions.

If travelling to areas where there are known infectious diseases, ballet companies must take extra precautions for all staff, including the necessary immunizations, personal hygiene training and making everyone aware of the risks. Because of the nature of a ballet company, with its close-knit community, intensity of physical training and proximity to each other, infectious diseases can spread rapidly. As a lot of dancers have a below average body weight, an infection and loss of more weight could have a really negative impact upon their muscles, their fitness and their recovery time. Seeking timely medical help is an essential step to prevent any further complications that may impact their career.

Modern Dance

In contrast to classical ballet, modern dance does not have such a specific set of technical and aesthetic boundaries. Often inspired by human emotions, much of modern choreography provides for greater freedom of movement and expression, challenging rather than simply entertaining the audience. There is no uniform image of perfection and the prettiness and etherealism of ballet are firmly rejected in favour of realism. It comes in a huge variety of styles and techniques, all reflecting individual attitudes towards the fundamental principles of movement. Consequently, the demands on the body can be very variable, as can the aesthetic and technical requirements of the dancer. Martha Graham, inspired by the human function of breathing, uses a ‘contraction and release’ technique which is further enhanced by the use of the floor in her choreography. Falling, rolling and kneeling, elements which are in direct contrast to ballet’s emphasis on ‘lift’ and high centre of gravity, may cause impact trauma to joints. Mark Morris on the other hand uses a lot of skipping and running in his choreography, characteristic of some types of folk dancing. Despite looking ‘easy’ and natural, the movements are incredibly energetic and fast-paced, with changes in direction and impetus. The risk of incorrect landings and transmission of force through the feet may cause lower limb injury. This chapter will now discuss some of these modern dance styles in more depth, how they developed over the years and their physical and psychological demands upon the body.

Technique

Modern dance technique emerged in the 1920s in rebellion against the 'artificiality' of ballet and its traditional, decorative movements. Over the decades, a vast array of different styles, techniques and dance purpose emerged; however, one aspect that unified all of these was the use of the body to express feelings through dance. The highly pointed foot, the constant turn out and the lengthened spine and high centre of gravity of ballet were no longer accepted as necessary foundations for movement. New foundations developed in antithesis to these balletic ideals: feet could be flexed or relaxed, and bare; hips could be in parallel or rotated inwards; the torso freely curving; and all parts of the body and the floor could be used. Modern dancers no longer had the ballerina's issue of squeezing feet into pointe shoes and worrying about bunions, ligament strains and ankle impingement. Nor the stresses of maintaining extreme levels of turnout and its associated risk of hip, knee and lower back problems. Their movements could be liberated from such 'unnatural', unrelenting standards. However, each of the modern styles we saw then and we see today, with their own defining movement characteristics, have their own set of physical demands and injury risk.

Martha Graham was a pioneer of modern dance and her style has influenced a wide range of modern choreographers over the years. The body's core is the foundation of her technique: contracting and curving the torso inwards, followed by a release, expanding the chest and arching the spine, often both combined with spiral twists. With a lot of force as is characteristic of her style, this can pressurize the spinal vertebrae and potentially lead to disc degeneration and back pain. Her movements are often violent and blunt, throwing the body around, thudding bare heels, dropping to the knees or falling onto the floor. Strenuous, pounding jumps and sharp body angles create this impression of struggle and effort of movement; the dancer is visibly battling with gravity, emphasizing our connection to the earth. The dancers themselves must be powerful and strong, otherwise joints will be strained. Without the cushioning effect of soft landings, the shock of impact on bones against the floor may result in serious damage, and the overall visual body tension required of the dancer will be incredibly draining, both physically and mentally.

In contrast, Merce Cunningham, another founder of the modern dance revolution, preferred his movements less weighted to the floor, with less concentrated emotion. Speed and dexterity were emphasized, with quick rhythmic footwork, lightly pointed feet and extended legs. The torso was used much more freely, to build momentum in brisk, darting jumps across the stage. This almost frantic movement style may be very strenuous on the cardiovascular system, as well as the feet and knees.

Some of the more post-modern dance styles may require minimal dance technique of any kind. The simplicity of choreography and economy of movement may in fact seem ordinary – which is often the goal. The dancers' movements often represent normal, everyday activities, resonating with the audience because they can relate to them. Instead of any set positions and movement boundaries associated with some of the earlier modern techniques, the dancers are instructed to listen to their bodies and move in relaxed, economical ways. All parts of the body can be used, from the eyes to individual toes and fingers. Improvisation may be a substantial part of the choreography, where the dancers can move in ways that feel most natural to them, perhaps highlighting their individual strengths. This release of tension and emphasis on going with the flow of movement puts much less strain on the body. Instead of fighting it, the dancer is working with it. However, because of the relative lack of technical training compared to ballet, the dancer may push themselves in undisciplined ways, unaware of the consequences. The feet may not be adequately strengthened to perform those turns and jumps, or the lumbar regions may be at risk from a lack of core strength and stability.

Interestingly, some other post-modern styles contrast completely with this, almost coming full circle and requiring dancers to have mastered the classical ballet technique. Indeed a lot of new choreography involves a melting pot of dance styles from all parts of the globe. Mark Morris likes to make his choreography as difficult for the dancer as possible. Rather than playing to the dancers' strengths, he will consciously challenge them, making right-turners turn left and slower movers to jump as fast as possible. The final result is unimportant; the way the dancer gets there is. Obviously, this might prove quite a physiological and emotional struggle as the dancer tries to work against their natural capabilities and movement instincts, with failure the overriding result.

This disregard for classical rules and hierarchies follows on into dance roles and partnering. The corps de ballet/soloist/principal structure of the large classical ballets is less apparent in modern works. One large group of dancers may carry a complete work, while other pieces may involve just a single dancer. Sometimes soloists may emerge from an ensemble, without any specific distinguishing characteristics or technical talents to separate them from the group. Rather than having a narrative role to play, they may just be fulfilling the choreographer's aesthetic vision. Often multiple dancers may be doing different things on stage at the same time, leaving room for the audience to choose who to watch. Furthermore, ballet's gender stereotyping is often turned on its head. Rather than the heroic prince supporting and protecting the delicate ballerina, dancing partnerships are explored from alternative angles where sex or gender are much less confined or indeed even considered. The potential for new shapes, angles and relationships between dancers is thoroughly exploited by modern choreographers. Both partners may perform virtually identical movements, or even swap steps completely. The female may lift or support the male, partner another female, and vice versa. Matthew Bourne's male Swan Lake includes stunningly athletic pas de deux work, where both qualities of strength and sensitivity are displayed in equal measure. However, with this new approach to partner work and the constant pushing of boundaries, injuries caused by risky lifts, counter balances and improvisation may be a real issue in modern dance companies. Females may be required to do additional strength training in order carry out lifts safely. Trust and sufficient technical preparation are key to contemporary choreography.

Training

Graham and Cunningham techniques are probably the most well-known among contemporary training styles, but unlike ballet, there is no collective school of thought. Some contemporary dancers may go through 3 or more years of full time vocational Cunningham training, alongside ballet classes, whilst others may have no formal training at all. Choreographers may want a dancer to move in a raw, free way that's not encumbered by technical precision and boundaries. As such, this could be both beneficial in terms of reducing undue repetitive, technical stresses on the body, but may also expose them to injury if their bodies are inadequately conditioned to perform.

If training in the Graham technique, a typical 'class' contrasts with ballet: instead of starting at the barre, the dancer begins a series of exercises sitting or rolling on the floor – placing quite a lot of pressure on protruding bones in the leaner dancer. Work then steadily progresses to standing and then travelling, again with much more emphasis on parallel work, flexed feet and alternate contractions/relaxations.

There is a lot more variety in contemporary dancer body-aesthetics. With such an array of styles, choreographic narrative and rebellion against the classical ideal, there is no prevalent 'perfect' body type, ethnicity or even age. Strength and movement ability are much more highly favoured than a long neck and high arches. This acceptance of individuality, with all a dancers strengths and weaknesses, creates a much healthier outlook, particularly for the younger dancer. There is much less pressure to conform to a potentially deleterious body image, as well as forcing the muscles, tendons and bones into uncompromising positions that the dancer may not have the facility for. With an all-encompassing attitude to race and colour, modern dance is much further ahead than ballet in creating a world where dancers are valued for their talent and their individuality rather than for pre-defined and rather archaic aesthetic parameters.

Other Styles of Dance

A detailed consideration of the many other styles of dance is beyond the scope of this chapter, but the reader should be able to predict many of the occupational risks to the musculoskeletal system by working through the principles outlined above.

Many dance styles reflect ethnic traditions and are therefore especially suited to the bodily characteristics of the appropriate ethnic groups. This might not just reflect height, weight and body build but can also have more subtle inferences. There is an ethnic variation in muscle structure and the proportion of fast and slow twitch muscle fibres in some racial groups, which might enhance or restrict the strength of the jump. There is also inherited racial variation in collagen structure which largely determines flexibility. Different ethnic dance styles are likely to play to these characteristics.

Even "European" dance styles hold surprises. Ballroom dancing might be considered the province of the elderly but the athleticism required for competitive ballroom dancing at an elite level is substantial, this level of the sport almost entirely restricted to younger people.

Chapter 4
The Voice and the Musculo-Skeletal System

Introduction

Management of the larynx and the adjacent parts of the airways falls into the province of the Ear, Nose and Throat specialist and technique is mainly the province of the vocal coach. Nevertheless it is often forgotten that singing also requires an efficient source of air production involving the integrity and efficient functioning of the chest, diaphragm an abdominal wall. In addition posture is important, not just involving the thoracic spine, but especially the cervical spine which determines the position of the head and voice projection. In turn the upright stance, lumbar spine and even the stability provided by the legs and feet are also of some importance.

This chapter briefly discusses the role of the laryngologist and also concentrates on the musculo-skeletal aspects of singing which are often neglected. Indeed there are very few parts of the body that do not play a part in the production of the singing or acting voice. Much of the information contained is also relevant to woodwind and brass players.

H.A. Bird, *Performing Arts Medicine in Clinical Practice*,
DOI 10.1007/978-3-319-12427-8_4,

The Thorax and Abdomen

The voice is powered by air exhaled from the lungs; the true bellows. They are passive organs within the thoracic cage, inflating on inspiration and deflating on expiration. They sit within the relatively rigid compartment created by the surrounding chest wall, the base of which is formed by the diaphragm, made up of muscle and fibrous tissue and the most flexible part of the cage. As it contracts it flattens, moving downwards, and draws air down through the larynx into the lungs. It then relaxes involuntarily such that air passes back out through the larynx passively, contraction of the ribs to produce additional exhalation contributing only a little (abdominal breathing). In singing voluntary active contraction of the muscles of the abdominal wall also occurs, pressing up against the diaphragm which acts like the plunger of a syringe, so the flow of air through the larynx is now controlled by the singer who may also invoke active movement of the chest wall to further enhance the flow of air.

Full assessment of the singer's air supply therefore includes the exclusion of lung disease and assessment of the phrenic nerve and abdominal musculature as well as the function of the ribs and thoracic spine.

The Larynx

This is most crucial structure for producing both speech and song and is shown intact from the back in Fig. 4.1. It is essentially a set of three valves or sphincters, designed to protect the lungs from the inhalation of food when food is swallowed. The lowest valve is the true vocal folds or cords, the airway between them called the glottis or glottis aperture. The muscular false (vestibular) vocal folds are a little above the glottis and form a second valve. The floppy cartilaginous epiglottis is above these and is the highest of the three valves. Figure 4.2 shows a dissected view of the larynx from the side, illustrating the relative positions of these three sphincters on their

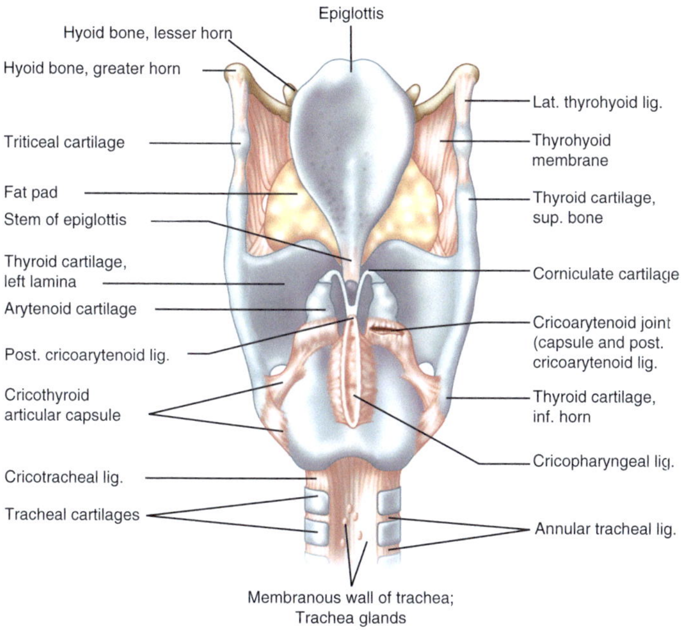

FIGURE 4.1 The intact larynx

cartilaginous scaffold. The whole apparatus also moves upwards during swallowing to confer further protection.

The part that is adapted for phonation, the glottis, comprises a pair of "curtains", the vocal cords, held in place across the airway by a cartilaginous frame made up of the thyroid and cricoid cartilages. They comprise thin strips of muscle and a ligament, covered by mucous membrane. They are shown, seen from above in Fig. 4.3. The true vocal cords appear white and the false vocal folds above them appear pink. They can be moved within the scaffold by a complex group of muscles, the intrinsic laryngeal muscles, which between them swivel and tip the small jug like arytenoid cartilages to which the cords are attached posteriorly. Figure 4.4 illustrates the actions of some of these muscles in opening and closing the vocal cords.

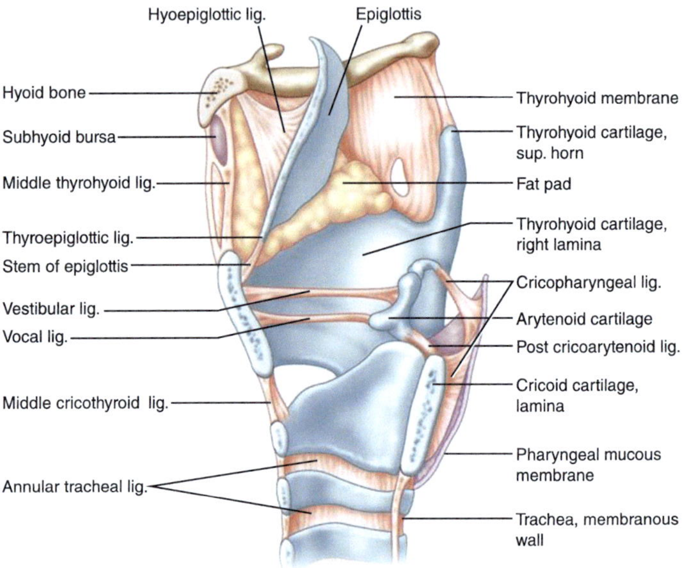

FIGURE 4.2 Dissected larynx in cross-section showing the cartilaginous scaffold

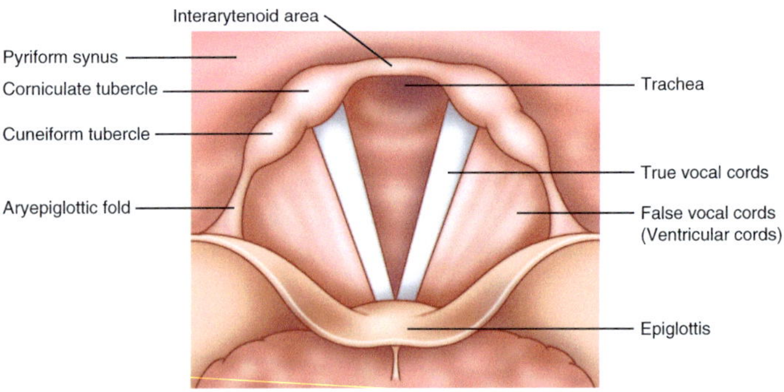

FIGURE 4.3 The vocal cords, seen from above

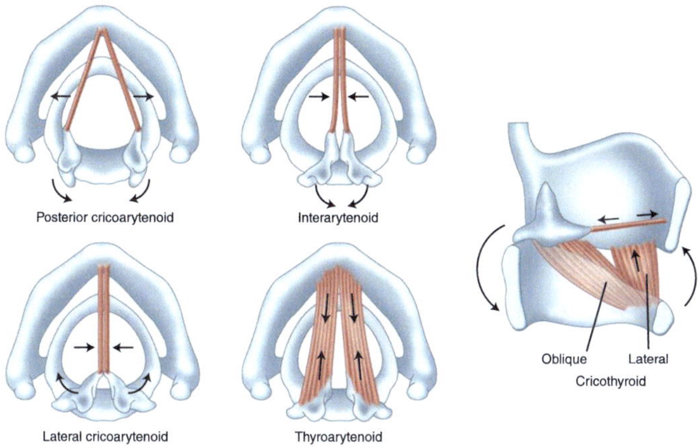

FIGURE 4.4 Actions of the intrinsic laryngeal muscles

Singing is achieved through a refined voluntary balance between the muscular tension that draws the folds together towards the closed position and the force of the subglottic air from below that pushes them apart. This sets the vocal cords, which actually more resemble floppy lips, vibrating hundreds of times a second to produce a sound. The tension in the folds is then controlled by complicated patterns of striated muscular contraction to define pitch. Aspects of this control have to be learnt. For example, with the soprano voice pitch in the upper part of the range is controlled by the cricothyroid muscle whereas in the lower part it is controlled by the vocalis and arytenoid muscles. Smooth transition from chest to head voice across "the break" is difficult and only achieved through practice.

Any suspicion of a disorder in this part of the vocal apparatus should prompt early referral to an expert laryngologist. Not only does a laryngologist have appropriate expertise; they also have access to specialized investigative techniques including laryngoscopy, nowadays quick, easy and invariably diagnostic.

Laryngeal Disorders

This is somewhat outside the author's rheumatological expertise and the reader is referred to more comprehensive texts listed in the bibliography.

Acute and chronic laryngitis can normally be diagnosed clinically but early expert referral is still advised because of more serious pathologies that may mimic these conditions. Such pathologies that are often found in singers and may be associated with the intensive use of their larynx that is required for their art form include vocal nodules, cysts of the vocal folds, vocal fold haemorrhage and laryngeal polyps. More serious pathologies such as cancer of the larynx can occur in anyone, even singers.

The Supralaryngeal Structures

These comprise the pharynx, nose, mouth, tongue and palate.

Once the basic sound is created in the larynx, it is subject to considerable further refined modification in the supralaryngeal structures which because their complexity as well as the further strictures, behave as a series of further air containing cavities, each of different shape and character and each acting as a resonator with the potential to modify the sound further. Moreover each of these resonators is capable of changing shape, some under neurological control. If the function of the pharynx is mainly involuntary and the nose fixed in contour, the tongue and height of the palate are very much under voluntary control. The sinuses, once thought to act as important resonators, may contribute only a little.

Finally, the lips, tongue tip and even the teeth achieve a final articulation before the sound finally produced reaches the listener's ear.

The human vocal apparatus has a total range of some five octaves across all singers from soprano to bass. Each individual will have their own personal range, some larger than others, determined partly by training but mainly by the anatomical characteristics of their body and to some extent their hormonal background.

The Trunk

Unlike most instrumentalists, singers normally perform in an erect position, facing and especially communicating with the audience. Their body is their instrument. Posture is therefore important.

The thoracic spine assists in air production and the lumbar spine provides a firm base for the abdominal apparatus, with counterbalance to the anterior abdominal wall. Minor musculoskeletal abnormalities in the chest, amongst them costochondritis can be crucial and minor degrees of scoliosis, typically casing slight inequality in shoulder height, will also affect function. Where a scoliosis also involves the lumbar spine, abdominal function may be impaired and the general erect stance, so important for communication, may be compromised. Additional musculoskeletal effort may be needed to maintain stability and posture if segments of the spine are hypermobile. The pelvis, legs and even feet all play a part in posture though in the dramatic singer or in opera, minor movements of the spine can be useful in enhancing dramatic effect.

Most important but often ignored is the cervical spine and the shoulder girdle. Muscles acting at these places also play a role in accessory respiration acting at the upper limit of the rib cage and displaced intervertebral discs can impinge on the phrenic nerve. The angle of the head, often important in communicating the meaning of a song and the freedom of the jaw both depend on efficient function of the topmost cervical vertebrae.

Ageing

Professional dancers peak early and often retire between the ages of 30 and 40, though in some countries, particularly those of Eastern Europe, there is a tendency to continue dancing until later, and this is often achieved anyway through a transition to less active forms of dance such as ballroom dancing. Instrumentalists tend to perform at the highest level for two or three decades longer and after continue to play at a high amateur standard. There is a strong impression that singers perform longer than anybody else, even after giving up a musical instrument, hence the brief consideration of ageing in this chapter.

However, any public perception that singing may be less susceptible to the biological effects of ageing is clearly incorrect. Various natural changes occur in the body with age.

Collagen, the basic biochemical building block of the body, which exists in many forms according to its exact location and purpose, stiffens with age through the mechanism of forming chemical crosslinks called disulphide bridges that reduce the capacity of the filaments to slide one upon another. So the flexibility and therefore the versatility of the larynx is reduced.

Cartilage, which in combination with synovial fluid, creates a bearing with a coefficient of friction less than ice on ice at articulating joints becomes worn with age, less smooth and later even fissured, partly through "wear and tear" but also because of biochemical changes inherent in ageing. The cartilage in the larynx, essentially an articulation, performs less efficiently.

Muscle bulk, normally maintained through exercise, may reduce whenever activity is reduced in the elderly as it often is. Neurological pathways become less efficient as a proportion of the neurons that make up the nerves atrophy with age, resulting in slight impairment in the neurological control of the muscle. So control of the larynx itself is less precise and the capacity of the bellows is reduced functionally.

This can lead to poorer breath control, loss of vocal stamina, some voice tremor and difficulty regulating pitch. There are also likely to be alterations in vocal range, normally a high voice becoming lower though this may in part be as much hormonal as ageing. Of the three main sex hormones, testosterone, oestrogen and progesterone, all three present in both sexes though in varying amounts according to gender, testosterone influences muscle bulk and function whilst progesterone has a relaxant effect on some sorts of collagen. In adolescence, because of hormones and growth, the treble range migrates downwards and in females the menopause introduces various changes to the voice.

Accomplished singers will have developed various tricks of technique to use their voice to maximum benefit, that can also be used to counteract some of the effects of ageing. In addition there is likely to be a change of repertoire away from less demanding roles. For example a change from opera to lieder will compensate for the less efficient bellows and needs less volume and projection of the voice.

Gerontologists also recognize a variation in the speed at which people age. So whilst some individuals will be “showing their years” others of exactly the same age and sex will seem “ever youthful”. Traditionally this was attributed to sociological factors, perhaps including wealth and even linked to intelligence. Recently it has become accepted that there is also a true genetic variation in the success of ageing, attributable to changes in the inherited chromosomes. This is thought to be related to inter-individual variation in telomere function. Telomeres clip the ends of chromosomes, analogous to the plastic tips of shoelaces. Each time throughout life that a cell and its chromosomes divide, a little chromosome material is lost so they become very slightly shorter and less efficient. In some genetically favoured individuals, telomeres are thought to be more efficient in reducing this wear.

Overall the social benefits of instrumental playing and singing and the exercise each can provide recommend continued participation in music strongly as a means of combating old age.

Case Study: A Singer with Musculoskeletal Problems

Introduction

His case study describes a singer who had problems with her technique that initially puzzled her singing teachers that were probably mainly attributable to musculo-skeletal problems that had not initially been noticed.

Case History

GC had been an enthusiastic soprano since the age of 6. Throughout her childhood and adolescence, no concerns had been raised by her singing teachers as she progressed through her graded examinations. By the time she left school to read music at university, with singing as her main subject, she was singing for around 6 h a week. On arrival at university, her new singing teacher drew her attention to tension in the neck, especially when she was singing her high notes. Towards the end of her first term it was considered that this was handicapping her progress and she was referred to a Performing Arts Medicine clinic.

She was first seen in December 2012, soon after her 18th birthday. On reflection she suspected the tension might have been present in a milder form for the previous 4 years though had not been an issue in her less demanding repertoire. If so this would have been an onset about 1 year after her menarche, though the problem was not cyclical in relation to her periods.

Specifically, the tension in the neck was aggravated only when she sang the top F of the stave and the notes above. It was especially aggravated by passages that jumped in and out of this range though she also considered that a further aggravating factor was when she had slept in an awkward position that had caused a "crick in the neck". After that the symptoms would be more pronounced, usually for some days. Her overall vocal range was from the F or even the E below the treble stave, up to the A above the treble stave.

On examination at a brief initial assessment the neck was indeed held stiffly, almost awkwardly, partly because she seemed to stretch it upwards in order to hit her high notes. Otherwise there was no obvious clinical abnormality in the musculo-skeletal system. Within the 30 min available for the appointment, posture appeared normal and the shoulder height was equal. Neurology was also normal on course testing.

An opinion was given that x-ray of the cervical spine initially and perhaps later the thoracic spine might be helpful.

She agreed to take a letter requesting these to her general practitioner during the vacation. Unfortunately, to her disappointment and that of her parents the doctor declined to arrange X-rays arguing that there was not sufficient clinical indication. The X-rays therefore had to be obtained in the private sector on her return to university.

A further appointment was then made of some 90 min with a vocal coach in attendance for a second opinion, at which the X-rays were also reviewed. These had been reported by the radiologist as excluding spinal disease with additional comment on "minor positional changes".

The suspicion had to be, however, that an interruption of the normal curve of the cervical sine at the C4/C5 level together with a possible slight compensated "S" shaped scoliosis between C5 and T5 might be relevant to her vocal problems (Figs. 4.5 and 4.6).

This impression was reinforced when she warmed up for 15 min and then sang varied repertoire for 30 min until pain occurred in the neck and her difficulty at the higher notes became most pronounced. By now there was also some pain in the left shoulder. Re-examination at this point now revealed a slight difference in shoulder height with the left shoulder slightly rotated forward compared to the right. At this point she conceded she often "self-manipulated" the spine to correct this twist when she was tired but had not previously connected it with her vocal problems.

Medical management was therefore with a "V-shaped" support pillow at night, and a trial period of singing with the left arm in a sling until conventional physiotherapy exercises together with Alexander Technique strengthened and stabilized the spine.

Musical management was to restrict singing to shorter but more frequent 20 min periods so the total amount of singing remained unaltered and to leave the main university choir which contributed little to her degree in favor of more time with her chamber and solo repertoire, which did.

An immediate issue for the degree course was the need to perform a 25 min baroque recital the same term. The

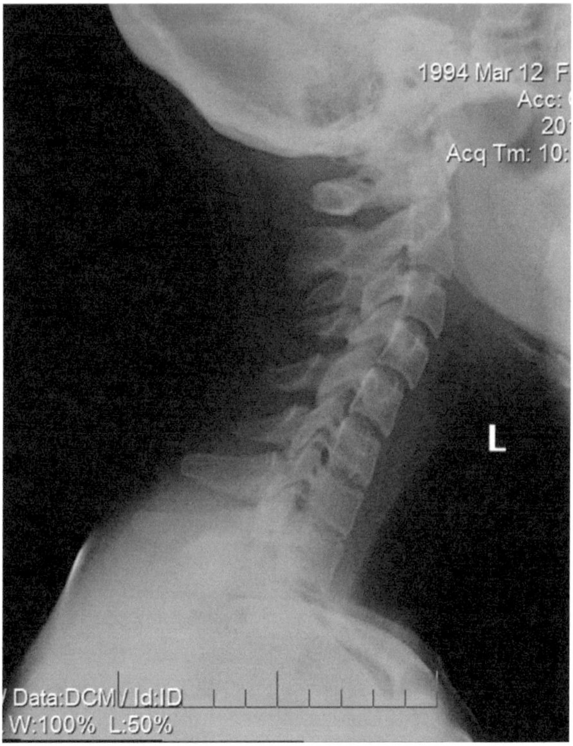

FIGURE 4.5 Cervical spine lateral view

programme for this was reviewed and on medical advice, one piece was substituted with another that did not strain her top notes so much. This proved perfectly acceptable to the university authorities.

Comment

This case illustrates the importance of always considering the musculo-skeletal system as a cause of vocal problems in a singer. Even though a brief initial examination was normal, the fact that vocal technique was especially impaired when the

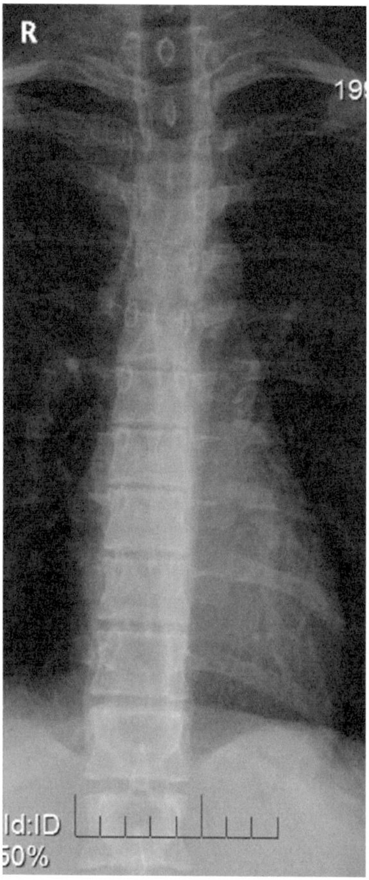

FIGURE 4.6 Thoracic spine PA view

neck was painful after sleeping in an awkward position had to provide a strong clue, sufficient to justify further investigation.

The second longer appointment, allowing the chance to sing different repertoire with a vocal coach in attendance, was then needed together with X-rays to fully clarify the problem and to plan treatment.

It was a disappointment that the General Practitioner declined to assist in treatment and the "normal" radiology report, when finally obtained, illustrates that most radiologists concentrate on excluding spinal disease without attention the clinical ergonomic factors around performance and the ways in which quite subtle variations in spinal structure can influence elite performance.

The longer 90 min appointment was invaluable in challenging the voice, almost to the point of fatigue, when new clinical signs became apparent.

Finally, the case illustrates that medical management is best complemented with attention to the repertoire and that quite small changes made to this can assist the immediate situation until the benefit of standard medical treatment becomes apparent.

Chapter 5
Principles of Management
Diagnosis, Treatment, Rehabilitation and Prevention

Introduction

This text does not seek to provide an encyclopaedia of the many different medical conditions that can afflict instrumentalists, dancers and vocalists. Excellent textbooks already exist for that and are listed in the biography at the end of this book. Rather it seeks to explain how Performing Arts Medicine differs from the many other branches of medicine, even Sports Medicine to which it is perhaps most closely related. It attempts to draw attention to practical points in management and ways of avoiding pitfalls that have plagued the author in his many years of self-tuition during which all his medical and rheumatological skills have been tested to the limit.

The full assessment and management of the elite professional performer, and even of the part-time amateur takes time. For the elite performer a full hour for an instrumentalist and even up to 2 h for a dancer might be required.

The instrumentalist should bring their own instrument whenever practical as well as any music that they consider is causing them difficulty so that this can be reviewed. Sometimes the instrument is too large to transport or the performer may have concern about exposing an instrument of value to a hospital environment. At times I have tried keeping both a cello and an electronic keyboard, substituting for a piano, in

H.A. Bird, *Performing Arts Medicine in Clinical Practice*,
DOI 10.1007/978-3-319-12427-8_5,

the consulting room but have found that these tend to miss clinical nuances that are revealed when the performer is using their own regular instrument.

An alternative is to conduct the clinic in a music school. Whilst this might require some improvisation of clinical facilities (though some conservatoires now boast a medical room), there are advantages in having access to sound-proof practice rooms containing a panoply of different larger instruments.

Similar considerations apply to dancers. The longer appointment time is not entirely related to their often greater complexity, but also to the fact that the dancer who is warmed up is a different creature to the dancer who is cold and some injury assessment may only be possible after warm-up or even on fatigue, usually after class. The arguments for assessment in or adjacent to a studio become stronger though even in a clinic there may be floor space for warm-up, perhaps in an adjacent empty room and either an examination couch (especially one of adjustable height) or a wall rail designed for the disabled can often serve as a ballet barre. Most dance conservatoires nowadays boast a physiotherapy treatment room that can serve for clinical examination.

Diagnosis

An accurate diagnosis is clearly essential and this is usually easier for the acute injury than for the complex long-term rehabilitation problem involving multiple sites. For many patients attending a Performing Arts clinic provisional, even definitive diagnosis has already been made, either at a local casualty department or by a physiotherapist, osteopath or chiropractor. Typically the performer has only sought help from or reached the specialist clinic because the problem has become chronic or more widespread.

Providing time allows, it is usually helpful to start with an instrumental or dance history. The elite instrumentalist usually has a single instrument though for some, for example percussionists, facility with several is required. The music student invariably has a main and a subsidiary instrument. Sometimes there are anatomical or physiological conflicts between the two. The amateur musician may enjoy playing several different instruments. Sports or hobbies that involve repetitive loading of the arms may impinge on the strains of music making. All of this "instrumental history" needs to be detailed, together with approximate milestones achieved, in a full assessment, since often a medical problem is unmasked by an instrument that is not the main one. It is also helpful to enquire which composers or which particular passages of music cause problems and why. Performers are always body aware and their theories on causation often prove correct even if they are sometimes a little diffident in expressing them.

The dance history also enquire about the milestones achieved with each of the many different styles of dance since dancers, except the most elite, tend to need to be more versatile in the variety of dance styles that they offer to secure employment. It is particularly important to consider sports and activities that might constitute cross training since these also can impinge on dance injuries.

Simple questions concerning equality of leg length and turnout and shoulder height provide clues to the spinal and pelvic anatomy and the dancers assessment of their flexibility, endurance and explosive power (as in height of jumps) provides the physiological background.

Only then follows the injury history and the examination. The many conventional and accepted medical diagnoses that might emerge are beyond the scope of this chapter and are available in textbooks elsewhere. They are likely to include, tenosynovitis, carpal tunnel syndrome, epicondylitis and shoulder as well as spinal diagnoses in musicians and stress fractures, enthesopathies, impingement syndromes and many more in dancers. For all of these conditions, accepted investigations to confirm the suspected diagnosis exist and should be provided.

Perhaps more important are many problems that do not fall so easily within conventional medicine but which may still be the correct and most appropriate diagnosis for the performer, however contentious. Two such examples of "Overuse Syndrome", less appropriately sometimes termed "RSI" when it affects the arm, and "Hypermobility Syndrome" are dealt with in the referenced Chaps. 6 and 7 respectively. Perhaps these just represent sophisticated terminology for saying that the performer is pushing their body to limits that nature never really intended for artistic effect.

Treatment

Once a diagnosis or diagnoses are decided and confirmed by appropriate tests, appropriate treatment can commence. For an accepted medical condition such as tenosynovitis or carpal tunnel, treatment is also accepted and can be delivered though where several options exist the most conservative should normally be selected first. For carpal tunnel, rest with splinting, even if believed to be effective may be impractical for the performer wanting a speedy return to work. In turn injection therapy with removal of the ergonomic cause should probably be considered before operation, which always carries risks in performers, though sometimes operative release, even with its slight risk Complex Regional Pain Syndrome that could end a musical career, is necessary, the risk worth taking.

Surgery to the weight bearing joints in the legs and to the spine in dancers is even more fraught with problems and the best orthopaedic surgeons involved with performers invariably display a conservative streak sine operation at one joint sometimes perpetuates a problem by placing strain on adjacent joints, especially in the spine. These arguments also apply to the foot though because this is such an important part of the dancers anatomy simple operations with few risks may be crucial in allowing continuation of a career.

Treatment in Performing Arts Medicine has some inherent difficulties. Because many specialist clinics have charitable status, therapeutic follow-up may not be possible whilst the primary care practitioner may be out of their depth if treatment does not work according to plan.

Treatment is also given by a variety of practitioners whom possess different skill mixes and work from different raining backgrounds. Close communication is essential if wires are not to get crossed, especially as most performers tour incessantly.

Finally, only a small proportion of performers are on regular contracts. Especially in the self-employed, there is a tremendous incentive to return to work as soon as possible, often before healing is complete. Small companies or music groups depend on their performers so may not have the incentive to allow adequate convalescence. Performers themselves often consider it their duty to return to work in spite of pain “for the sake of their art”.

Rehabilitation

This important aspect is invariably neglected, largely because of the same constraints listed above that also apply to treatment.

For a simple injury, ideally decisions on speed of return to work should involve all practitioners as well as the performer and relevant administrator. The cause of the injury should be assessed as to whether it was a simple unavoidable accident or whether it arose from a fault in technique because the performer was attempting movements that were not appropriate to their physique or even because of local factors, for example a steeply raked stage. If an alternative performer can not be substituted changes in the musical repertoire or choreography may be needed until rehabilitation is complete.

For the more complex regional or chronic problems so often encountered in Performing Arts clinics, a longer period of rehabilitation is likely to be required. A return to the art form is likely to be gradual and graded. Musical repertoire or choreography should be selected with care and initially adapted where necessary although ultimately it may be desirable to re-challenge with the offending piece once technique has been improved.

Both for musicians and dancers some degree of parallel support or cross-training may be helpful. This might involve Alexander or Feldenkrais technique for musicians and Pilates or Yoga for dancers. Care should be taken to avoid sports that might aggravate during rehabilitation and it may be desirable to temporarily stop playing a second instrument to ensure there is only one instrumental variable as improvement is monitored.

Prevention

This falls into several categories.

For some acute injuries there is an obvious cause that could and perhaps should have been prevented even though it might not always have been appreciated by management.

For dance, one obvious example amongst many that could be cited from the authors experience is the problem of a costume designer who produces an overelaborate heavy headdress which the dancer has to wear while executing the steps required by the choreographer, leading to neck injury, especially with pirouettes. Another issue is lighting that is altered between rehearsal and performance so the option of spotting on a distant object is lost leading to loss of balance and injury. More subtle is the rake or angle of slope of the stage which varies between theatres so represents a hazard leading to foot injury if a touring company has not rehearsed on stages of different slope.

Such examples are less common in music though touring opera companies can encounter problems with the varying contours and size of the many different orchestral pits in which their orchestra is required to play. Similar problems may occur when a musical production moves to a smaller theatre.

It is a matter of debate whether all musicians should be able to play all music through improvement in their technique or whether some bodily characteristics will always cause difficulty with the music of certain composers. This author holds the latter view, especially in relation to pianists. Those composers who performed their own piano works invariably wrote music that mirrored the shape of their hands. Some composers such as Liszt and Rachmaninoff require large hands; Mozart can be played with much smaller hands. Crucially Rachmaninoff also had extraordinary lateral laxity of the middle digits of his hands and pianists who do not have this attribute tend to be more susceptible to overuse if they attempt to play his works. Clearly the composer is not now able to re-write them to help the performer.

There might be greater agreement with the suggestion that not all dancer's bodies are equally suited to the many different dance styles they might encounter. A good choreographer will adjust the choreography to suit the dancers available and some dancers might inspire choreography especially for them. Problems then occur when a second cast attempts the same piece, perhaps some time later, when the choreographer is no longer available to adjust the choreography to assist the body characteristics of the new dancers.

It goes without saying that good technique is crucial and can go a long way to preventing injury. For dancers and even musicians, this implies attention to warm-up with a general warm-up and then one more specific to the needs of the piece. Stretching exercises and cool down may be helpful as well as a gradual build up after periods of holiday and absence. Aerobic and cardio-fitness training may be useful, especially for dance. Different ethnic groups may benefit from training specifically targeting their ethnic attributes.

Ultimately, there could even be an argument that the choice of an instrument or particular dance genre, prior to commencing training, should be based on the performers anatomical and physiological characteristics, as might be customary in the world of elite sport. In turn training opportunities might be prioritized towards those most suited to benefit from them. The reasons for selecting an instrument or preferring a favourite style of dance are complex and this author is against selection on physical attributes alone. Nevertheless, if the clinician considers a performer is badly matched to their instrument, they perhaps have an obligation to point out that life might be more injury free with an alternative instrument. Ultimately, however, the performer must have the final say in their selection.

Chapter 6
Illustrative Case Histories: String Players with Multiple Problems

A Violinist with Multiple Musculoskeletal Problems

Introduction

This case history of an elite violinist provides an example of fortitude in overcoming multiple serial medical problems, almost all of which affected her playing. As so often, her return to serious violin playing required an integration of medical issues with the most appropriate repertoire and careful ergonomic analysis invariably revealed a rational cause for symptoms previously labeled as psychosomatic. She also provides testimony to the "cross-training" that can benefit musicians just as much as dancers.

Case History

AM, a Swiss violinist, self-referred to the author after attending one of his lectures given to the Science of Music postgraduate degree course at a major UK conservatoire where she was enrolled as a masters student in performance. She hoped that a combination of the medical content of the lecture, with insight from her father who was a gastroenterologist, would assist with her diagnoses, both past and present,

H.A. Bird, *Performing Arts Medicine in Clinical Practice*,
DOI 10.1007/978-3-319-12427-8_6,

which had sometimes been lacking from clinicians without knowledge of Performing Arts Medicine. Now aged 26, she had played the violin since infancy.

As a child she had always been talented, even precocious, and had therefore had a variety of teachers. She considered, probably correctly, that some of these might have pushed her too far too early in pursuit of their own fame. Because she had been experiencing musculo-skeletal problems since the age of 15, she initially rejected a career as a violinist such that her first degree was in French Literature. Postgraduate, she continued her studies in the USA where she was persuaded to return to her violin.

When first seen, she still aspired to be a professional soloist but sought an opinion on whether she might reasonably achieve this, given that the amount of playing required on her new performers course had already caused an exacerbation of her symptoms.

The previous history was sometimes a little difficult to interpret although she was an accurate and precise witness. The first event at the age of 15 she described as an "infected bursa" affecting the index finger of the right (bowing) arm. This was removed surgically but for a further 2 years she continued to experience symptoms and signs compatible with a tenosynovitis affecting the extensor tendons to the index finger as well as the thumb in the right hand.

When at the age of 19, both shoulders became stiff and sore after long periods of playing, she gave up the violin for a full year and studied French Literature at university. A convincing tennis elbow followed at the age of 20 attributed to her computer or perhaps to sport since she was now no longer playing the violin. At age 21 a neurologist diagnosed Carpal Tunnel Syndrome after nerve conduction studies. It was treated conservatively but by now she was becoming rather depressed. She said that psychosomatic illness was raised though it is hard to see on what grounds.

At the age of 23 she developed back pain localized to two sites, at T12 and at L5. At the age of 24 she prolapsed a lumbar disc at which stage a slight scoliosis was noted. Although her father requested imaging at this stage, this was denied her by a rheumatologist in Switzerland.

She had always considered herself sporty and was especially talented at horse-riding and ballet but gave this all up at the age of 15 for fear of interfering with her violin. When she had to give up her violin she had returned to some sports and ballet, also experimenting with martial arts and Pilates. She also enjoyed stretching to improve her mobility.

The only written medical opinion easily available was from a Sports Physiotherapist in the USA, dated May 2011, who she had seen for back pain. Perhaps as a result the report dwelt on a functionally shorter right leg and an inequality in shoulder height with some hyperextension of the spine at L5 though she was not obviously hypermobile elsewhere.

Two years before she was first seen by the author in February 2013, she had returned cautiously to her violin, still her main love, for up to 3 h a day. She still struggled with pain in the back and shoulders, often resorting to pain-killers. Of the many other treatment modalities she had tried, she felt that Alexander Technique and Tai Chi were the only two that had helped. Her dilemma was that after 9 years of symptoms, she would shortly need to avail herself of the opportunity to increase from 3 to 6 h practicing a day to achieve her aim of a career as a soloist. Given the less arduous alternatives of chamber music, orchestral rank and file or even teaching, she needed an urgent opinion on which of these she should aim for. She was reluctant to abandon the violin for her second instrument which was voice.

On a first brief examination in February 2013 the main features seemed to be that the right shoulder was held slightly lower than the left and was rotated forward. There was also some internal rotation of that shoulder that restricted the range of movement of the right upper arm. If she concentrated, she was able to "reset" this to give a more functional position for the right arm.

There was a difference between the two sides for lateral flexion of the lumbar spine though rotation was almost equal. There was, however, slightly greater turn-out at the right leg compared to the left and a slight difference in leg length.

Other aspects of the musculo-skeletal system were normal with no recurrence of any of the teenage aliments. Neurology also was normal to course testing.

She then played. Since a major recital was required from her by June 2013, after warm up she played samples of her proposed programme which was the Brahms second sonata, Chausson's Poeme and the Ravel Tzigane with a Paganini caprice and/or solo Bach in reserve. It was apparent that symptoms did not result from the style of a single composer as sometimes occurs.

Within minutes of starting to play the jaw tightened and as a result the neck became tense. Her strong suspicion was that her violin rest was a little too short for her long neck. Figures 6.1 and 6.2 show an example of a chin rest and how it is attached to the violin. Some further minutes later back discomfort occurred, localised to T12 and to L5. Even later the left shoulder tensed, which she said would be the precursor of paraesthesiae in the hand, possibly as a result of nerve root compression in the neck, though this was not formally tested.

She was reassured that her symptoms seemed not to be psychological and advised to concentrate on conventional back care with a firm mattress and a pillow that provided adequate support for the neck at night. Physiotherapy of the intensity and quality needed was not really an option with her timetable but she was encouraged to consider "cross-training", perhaps with the Tai Chi that had helped in the past. She was advised on a rational approach to the reduction of analgesics and allowed to proceed cautiously to longer periods of practice.

At follow up in March 2013 things were proceeding as planned. On examination it was now clearer that in addition to the features at the right shoulder noted before, the left lower rib cage was more prominent than the right, possibly causing the right shoulder to be lower, and that the left side of the pelvis was higher than the right.

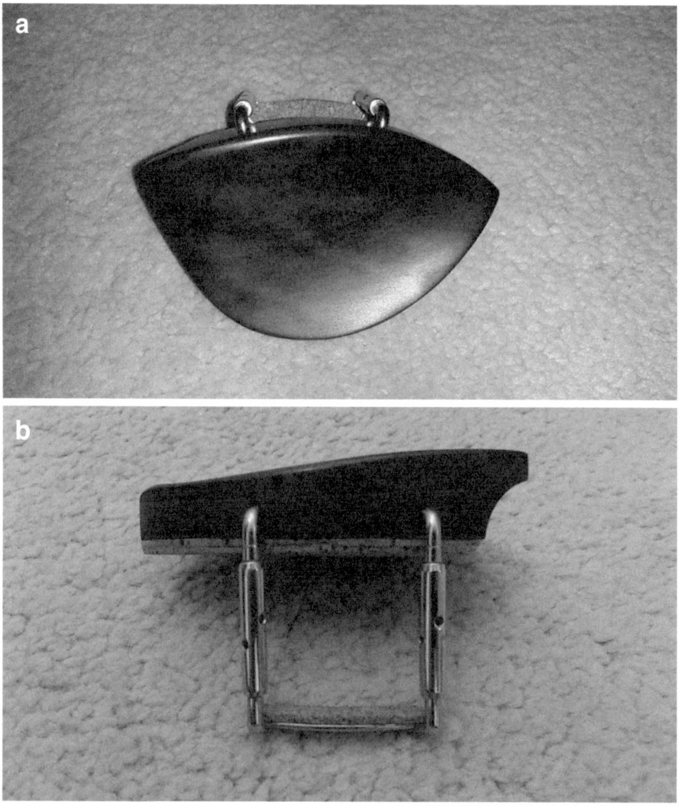

FIGURE 6.1 (**a**, **b**) Chin rest

At further follow up in August 2013, the recital had gone well and she was now playing for around 5 h a day without new symptoms or recurrence of old ones. She had followed the advice of teachers who encouraged her to play more freely with movement, rather than the advice of teachers who asked her to stand rigid. As a result she adjusted, even "self-manipulated" the spine to give relief when required, which in turn helped both neck and shoulders. She was now concentrating on Pilates rather than Alexander Technique which she felt to be more beneficial to the spine.

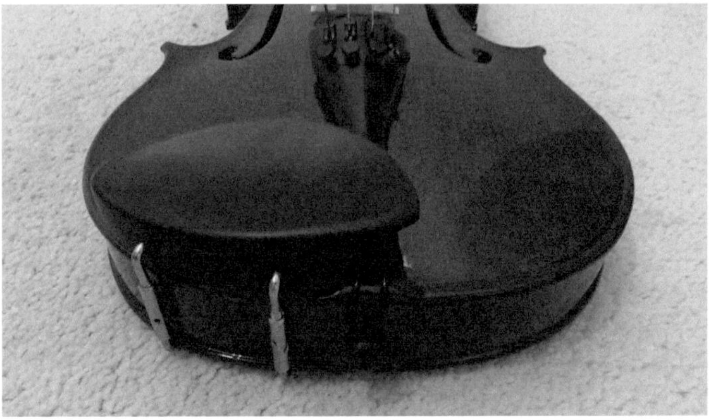

FIGURE 6.2 Attachment of chin rest

At further e-mail follow up in February 2014 she was comfortable playing all styles of music for almost 6 h a day, was spending an hour a day at Pilates and was sleeping on a firmer mattress. She still aspired to a solo career, the years already lost perhaps the main constraint.

Comment

This violinist was either very unlucky with her multitude of musculo-skeletal problems or perhaps fell into the category of clustering of problems within an individual. It is debated whether this is a discrete genetic entity or whether a pathology at one site might place extra ergonomic strain on an adjacent site, causing failure there too. Perhaps more plausible is the suspicion of a single predisposing factor, in her case the mild scoliosis, which still awaits confirmation on X-ray but which has been apparent on clinical grounds each time it has been looked for.

It is sometimes debated whether such a scoliosis is genetic or whether it is largely functional, created by the playing of an asymmetric instrument for up to 6 h a day throughout adolescence. Certainly the features observed at the shoulders might be a function of this but the features at the lumbar spine surely suggest a genetic aetiology throughout the spinal length. The patient preferred not to proceed to imaging to clinch the matter, and that view was respected.

It is disappointing that the suggestion of psychosomatic illness was made to account for her pain, when all of her symptoms were so easily explained in terms of the biomechanics in this elite performer. This did much to destroy her confidence and probably contributed to her decisions to leave the violin for extended periods to the probably detriment of her solo career.

A Double Bass Player with Multiple Problems Affecting the Upper Limbs

Introduction

This case illustrates a variety of upper limb problems that occurred in a professional orchestral double bass player, together with the strategies used to deal with each of them, culminating in an episode of sesamoiditis, with instructive inferences for its aetiology.

Case History

CS, a professional double bass player with the Opera North orchestra, was first seen at the request of the orchestral management in 2008 when she was aged 43. She was tall and had commenced playing the double bass at the age of 17. Apart from some minor issues of pain in the left shoulder around the age of 35, which she attributed, probably correctly, to overuse as she stretched the arm down the strings, she declared no major musculo-skeletal problems. These symptoms had responded to pacing herself and to conventional physiotherapy. She was right handed (her bowing arm).

She has been seen over a period of some 5 years in three main episodes, the first a recurrence of the left shoulder problem, the second with two separate injuries to the right thumb an the third with symptoms at the base of the little finger of the left hand, the more crucial hand in a bass player.

Episode One

In February 2008, towards the end of the winter season of operas, she was referred to a Performing Arts clinic with a recurrence of symptoms at her left shoulder which had been symptom free since her previous symptoms there resolved some 7 years earlier. She was one of only three permanent bass players employed by the orchestra. She had experienced aching at the left shoulder, at which a wide range of movement is required in bass players, sometimes radiating down the arm and worse towards the end of an opera. She had no symptoms in the right shoulder. She considered that the recurrence probably resulted the current repertoire since symptoms had worsened during the season. She further considered that this was probably because the three operas n the current repertoire, Peter Grimes, Madam Butterfly and Pinocchio, were particularly demanding on the bass section.

On examination, the left shoulder had a full range of movement and was pain free on examination early in the morning. There was no clinical evidence of an impingement or rotator cuff syndrome. There was no evidence of tenosynovitis or epicondylitis in the left arm. Neurological examination was normal with no evidence of carpal tunnel syndrome or nerve root compression. Movements of the neck were normal and pain free. There was, however a slight difference in leg length.

She was reassured that this was probably an overuse syndrome and that with appropriate pacing, perhaps also with physiotherapy of the sort that had helped her before, symptoms were likely to resolve once the operatic repertoire changed. The orchestral management was also sympathetic to spreading the load around the bass section as much as was possible. Symptoms did indeed improve with the advent of the new Spring repertoire.

Episode Two

In January 2009 she returned to the clinic with an injury to the right thumb. When her double bass was accidentally knocked from the side, in attempting to prevent it falling to the ground, she stretched out her hand and took the considerable weight of the instrument on the tip her right thumb. An X-ray of the thumb was normal and the injury healed over some 6 weeks as expected, the slow recovery probably attributable to her continued playing.

Unfortunately on the last day of a skiing holiday in March 2009, she suffered a passive hyperextension injury to the same thumb which caused immediate swelling and pain. A second X-ray was normal but ultrasound was also suggestive of a tear of the ulnar collateral ligament of the thumb with a small degree of synovitis in the metacarpo-phalangeal joint itself. Blood tests failed to show an evidence of auto-immune synovial disease and the synovitis was assumed to be traumatic in aetiology.

The right thumb is the less crucial thumb in a bass player but it was still necessary to adapt the position of the thumb on the bow and to stabilize it using a variety of aids. She tried several but found Lycra gloves to be the best with their combination of the support and flexibility required when she played . By contrast Glacier gloves and Futura wrist splints were too rigid though night resting splints were also of some value, improving symptoms the next day if worn on the night after a particularly long opera. A surgical opinion was also sought but in view of her adaption with the Lycra splint, surgical repair of the tear was not recommended.

She estimated that it took a full year before she was symptom free and was able to discard the Lycra gloves. This slow healing was also partly attributed to the fact that the company was embarking on the first opera of Wagner's Ring, with its demanding bass part.

Episode Three

She returned to the clinic in February 2013, some 4 years after the previous episode, again at the request of an enlightened orchestral management. There was now a problem at the base of the little finger of the left hand, the more important of the two hands in bass players and the little finger the smallest and therefore most fragile of the fingers in respect of the considerable pressure that it is required to exert on the heavy strings of the largest of all stringed instruments. The symptoms had been present for about 3 months. In the opinion of the player, this coincided with two operas, Othello and Die Walkure, simultaneously in repertoire, which represented the greatest challenge of the previous 4 years for the bass section.

Initially she experienced a sudden discrete swelling at the base of the left little finger during the 90 min third act of the third performance of Die Walkure. Within an hour of the end of the opera, swelling and erythema had radiated up the forearm for some 3–4 inches along the line of the tendons to the little finger. The general Practitioner, the next day, felt that the tendon was not infected and, reasonably, diagnosed tenosynovitis.

When see in the specialist clinic, 2 weeks later, after a period of relative rest, though not complete cessation of playing, the erythema and swelling along the line of the tendon was no longer present. There was, however, slight swelling at the metacarpo-phalangeal joint of the left little finger which was also tender to direct palpation. Otherwise, there were no clinical signs to support a diagnosis of auto-immune inflammatory arthritis or of degenerative change or of crystal deposition. There were some features of mild Raynaulds phenomenon and for the first time some mild joint hyperlaxity was noticed in the joints of the little finger. Now also under the care of her local rheumatologist, an ultrasound scan was arranged.

This showed a normal metacarpo-phalangeal joint and normal flexor and extensor tendons acting about that joint. However, there was a sesamoid bone adjacent to the joint over its ulnar aspect which was of irregular contour and of low echogenicity. These are more the features of a sesamoiditis rather than a fracture of the sesamoid bone.

Two surgical opinions were sought. Both recommended conservative management and with the use of ring splints (Fig. 6.3), she was once again able to continue playing. The function of the finger was reviewed with her instrument. Although there was no overt hyperlaxity of the joint at rest, when she demonstrated the intense pressure required of that

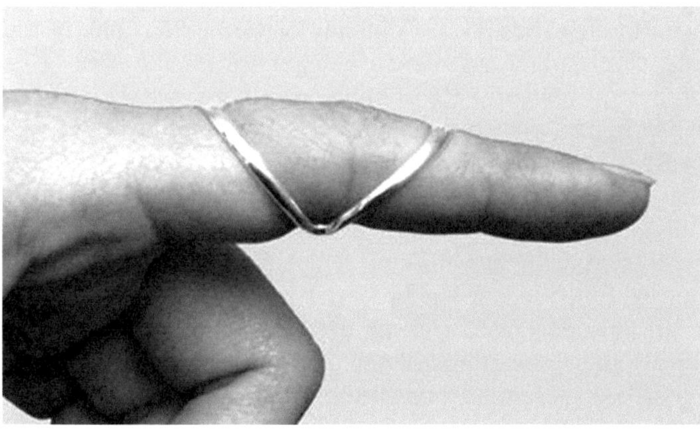

FIGURE 6.3 Ring splint in use

finger in playing Wagner, the joint did indeed become slightly unstable under pressure.

Comment

The case illustrates the value of a careful history with the practitioner prepared to pay full attention to the patients suggestions on causation and even changes required in technique to remedy the situation. Musicians and dancers are invariably "body-aware", intelligent and have a comprehensive training in technique. All that is needed is a practitioner, perhaps with some knowledge of the genre, to integrate this with medical pathology. In this case the "repertoire history" was a crucial as the conventional medical history.

It also emphasizes the need to consider and appreciate the asymmetry of the instrument concerned.

In episode two, the decision to allow the ulnar collateral ligament of the thumb to heal by natural conservative means, rather than by surgery, was a difficult one, particularly as the patient was allowed to continue with her playing, albeit with the injury affecting her less crucial thumb. Conventional immobilisation in a spica plaster for some 4–6 weeks would have prevented playing with its concerns for job security, even though the Opera Company concerned has one of the best records amongst Opera Companies for the care of its orchestral players. Reasonably, surgeons specializing in Performing Arts are reluctant to operate while there is a prospect of healing without surgery and this case vindicates that strategy. The downside is that complete healing took a full 12 months, but the patient was able to continue in her profession with her normal repertoire, subsequently with normal function, and the orchestra was not inconvenienced.

In episode three, it is suspected that the pathology was always the sesamoiditis rather than the tenosynovitis that it mimicked. Sesamoid bones are small bones embedded in tendons. The largest in the body is the patella in the quadriceps tendon and the pisiform at the wrist is another. At some sites they occur more variably, for example in the foot and less frequently in the hand. Their function is debated but those that are variable probably strengthen tendons, perhaps in response to repeated stress, even acting as a small pulley to allow the tendon to exert more power in its action. Those adjacent to the big toe often become inflamed, sometimes fractured, in dancers.

Symptomatic sesamoid bones are only occasionally encountered in musicians, but if only one site could be selected on ergonomic grounds, it would surely be in the left little finger in a double bass player, the inflammation possible precipitated by the particular repertoire at that time.

This dedicated performer took great trouble to research and evaluate a variety of aids that allowed her to continue with her playing and all the clinicians concerned learnt a lot from her experience and comments.

Chapter 7
Illustrative Case Histories: Dancers with Inflammatory and Degenerative Arthritis

A Dancer with Rheumatoid Arthritis; The Role for Biologics

Introduction

Inflammatory polyarthritis would normally be regarded as a contraindication to dance. However, treatment with new biological therapies may produce a more optimistic outlook even in this most arduous and competitive of professions. We here describe how one of us (AB) developed acute onset rheumatoid disease whilst a dance student and her resultant progress with modern drug therapy.

Case History

AB, born in 1986, commenced dance at the age of 12 years but only took it up seriously from the age of 16 years. Prior to this she had excelled at football, bandy (a precursor of ice hockey) and badminton in her native Sweden. From the age of 16 years she concentrated on contemporary ballet and African traditional dance as well as physical theatre. She considered herself less flexible than the average dancer but had good endurance and significant strength.

H.A. Bird, *Performing Arts Medicine in Clinical Practice*,
DOI 10.1007/978-3-319-12427-8_7,

After obtaining various awards in her own country, she was awarded a scholarship to study dance at Trinity-Laban Conservatoire for Music and Dance, an elite conservatoire in the United Kingdom. It was while she was attending physiotherapy there that she developed a sudden new onset of joint symptoms at the age of 23 years and the author was asked to see her by the superintendent physiotherapist. There was a strong suspicion from her symptoms and clinical signs that she had developed acute inflammatory arthritis. Referral was recommended, both to her general practitioner and to a rheumatology clinic. Arrangements were also made to see her again 2 months later at the conservatoire. From then on clinical care was managed jointly between her general practitioner, her local consultant rheumatologist and the author because of his interest in Performing Arts Medicine.

The initial symptoms had been pain and stiffness in the hands and feet, the pain in the feet particularly aggravated by the dancing. There was intermittent swelling in the hands and feet though initially no involvement of the wrists, elbows or knees. Initial management was with non-steroid anti-inflammatory drugs, mainly ibuprofen.

Within 6 weeks she was referred back to her local consultant rheumatologist when acute phase reactants were found to be slightly raised and rheumatoid factor was positive. She was commenced on methotrexate 25 mg a week as well as on hydroxychloroquine 200 mg a day, alongside her anti-inflammatory drugs. Folic acid supplementation was provided and depot injections of methotrexate were added.

Throughout this period she continued with her dance training. At intermittent review with the author on his visits to the conservatoire, the movements that were required for her continued training were reviewed, given her intended aim of completing her exams both in contemporary dance and ballet for contemporary dance. Artistically she had always found contemporary dance easier and more interesting than ballet.

In general the inflammation in the hands and feet was kept in control. An early problem was a spread of inflammation to both wrists and in contemporary dance often the weight of the body is taken on the wrists because of the floor work that is required. Her mother, who was an assisting occupational therapist and health consultant, provided guidance on splints through her colleagues and ways were devised of taking the weight of the body on other parts of the wrists that appeared not to be clinically affected. Throughout this period, reassuringly, there was no hint of flexion contracture either at the elbows or the knees.

She found the dancing increasingly difficult and an increase in the dose of methotrexate was prevented because of side effects. A case was therefore made for the early commencement of a biological agent and etanercept, in a dose of 50 mg subcutaneously each week, was selected following special funding from her local health authority. Methotrexate was continued alongside, now in a lower dose of 15 mg weekly as well as the folic acid.

There was considerable improvement following the introduction of etanercept allowing intra-articular steroid injections still to be held mainly in reserve and only used to control difficult flares of her arthritis.

However, a major problem arose in that the school timetabling required her to complete her ballet class early each morning when, inevitably, the diurnal variation in her rheumatoid disease caused the inflammation to be at its worst. Initially teachers were unable to comprehend why she should be so symptomatic early in the morning in the type of dance to which she was least suited, when she improved so much for her favourite contemporary classes later in the day. The diurnal variation, which had not previously been appreciated by the school, was explained. It proved impractical to re-schedule the ballet classes to later in the day so she was excused these, her examination assessment judged from her performance records before she had developed arthritis.

She was, however, able to continue with her course in contemporary dance with the help of the parallel discipline of Ashtangar Yoga, which although appearing severe, was well

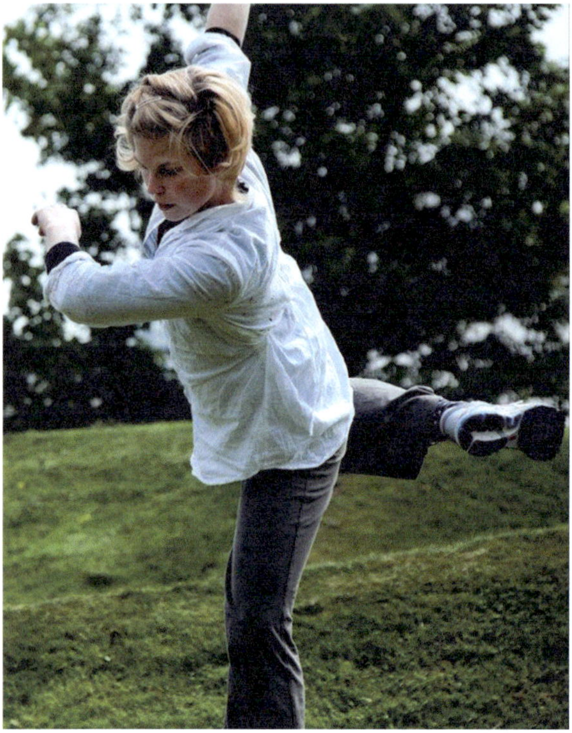

FIGURE 7.1 Dancing after treatment

taught and actually improved symptoms in her joints significantly.

To her credit she therefore completed her degree course with the help of etanercept combined with this careful guidance and has since continued to dance (Figs. 7.1 and 7.2).

Subsequently, she spent some time selecting the most suitable career path and most recently was working in a job that combined some dance with choreography, teaching and marketing at a company (Candoco Dance Company) that specialises in employing and integrating disabled and non-disabled dancers. This company was founded by Celeste Dandeker who had herself been rendered paraplegic by a fall on stage while dancing.

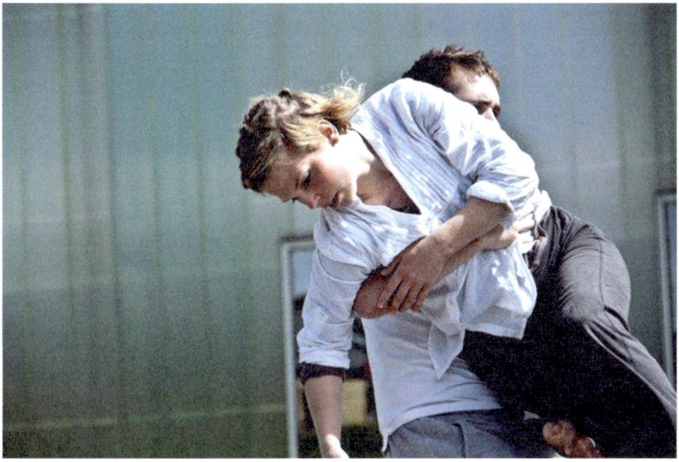

FIGURE 7.2 After treatment. There is no evidence of active synovitis at the hands or wrists

Discussion

This case history illustrates what can be achieved with close collaboration between several experts. These here comprised her general practitioner, the physiotherapist, a consultant rheumatologist, a rheumatologist specialising in performing arts medicine and the patient's mother who was an occupational therapy assistant providing advice from a country (Sweden) where high taxation allows the highest standards of medical care and rehabilitation.

The dancer herself also displayed considerable enterprise in learning about her disease such that she was largely able to predict which joints might normally be affected next and to take preventative action. This invariably involved modification of her technique with adapted movements that eased the ergonomic strain on the joints.

The lack of appreciation that certain styles of dance could be much more demanding in this individual than others and the lack of appreciation of the natural diurnal variation in inflammatory arthritis initially caused considerable misunderstanding that required careful explanation and rectification.

Overall, the hands and feet, normally the joints most severely affected in rheumatoid disease, proved surprisingly unproblematic even in a dancer. The wrists became more of a problem especially when she was unable to move them into the optimum position to take the weight of the body on the hands. In that the ankles also became problematic, it is possible that these joints were used excessively to compensate for her instinctive protection of the feet. Her yoga exercises were modified to guard against typical problems of rheumatoid disease such as flexion contracture at the knees and she devised a completely new warm-up to meet her needs, which she said she needed to change from month to month. This required longer time than a normal warm-up, especially early in the morning.

It also became necessary to work closely with the dance school authorities. Her scholarship did not cover all of the ever-increasing fees such that for parts of her training she had to take an evening job, which was essential financially but which added to the ergonomic strain placed upon her joints, particularly the wrists.

The Patients Viewpoint

One of the most difficult things in facing Rheumatoid Arthritis was realising that the body I had once known and learnt how to master for 23 years were no longer there, or at least not in the way it used to be. Being a dancer and a performer I have got to know my body very well as the profession demands the constant presence of every inch of my physical and mental body. As a dance practitioner this has always been my objective to be fully cognizant and to always deliver everything that I do whole-heartedly.

When I fell ill I could no longer sense every inch of my body, it was "blocked" by pain and inflammation. My sense of orientation in the studio and on stage was decreased and so was my ability to move. It proved very difficult to do everyday tasks such as eating, holding a pen or having a shower. All these things were of course frightening and difficult to accept.

I could have given up my profession and passion there and then but I did not. I am a person that does not give up easily, and for better and for worse, I am a fighter and decided to find my way through it. I was grateful to meet doctors who could help me and who also wanted to find a way forward and encouraged me to continue in dance. They helped me with their medical expertise so that I could also keep hold of my own faith and belief that there is a way to live with a rheumatic disease and still have a career within the world of dance.

It has been a struggle and a tough journey during these first 3 years with Rheumatoid Arthritis, filled with grief, pride and joy.

Now, I can accept that it is not a case of losing the body I once had, but that my body has changed. With regards to the grief that I have experienced for lost dreams, it has become clear that as much as anything this had to do with me developing my own sense of self esteem and my wish to build a sustainable career.

I am proud that I worked and am succeeding in turning things around, making things possible and helping others on the way. Not only did I fight to finish my degree at the conservatoire, I also did it for the students coming after me to prove that it is possible to dance despite physical impairment. I never thought I would finish my studies but I did, and the very same spring I managed to climb Ben Nevis with some wonderful help and support from friends, also proving the impossible to be possible.

When I started on Etanercept I was able to enjoy dancing again after only a few months of being on the new drug. During this time I found that the pain eased, the inflammation calmed down and the physical connectivity of my body improved. As the pain became more bearable I was able to start building strength again to support myself and slowly but surely got better. Most importantly the change helped me believe that it was possible to turn things around and that I was able to make the change happen. In my view, a sense of belief is crucial when one is fighting an attack on ones own body, as the attack can easily, and often does, make you feel helpless.

I continue working with and managing my condition with the disciplines of Pilates, Yoga and Hydrotherapy, alongside continued treatment with Etanercept, Leflunomide (substituting for Methotrexate because of the side effects caused by that drug required reduction to a sub therapeutic dose) and Ketoprofen.

The combination of my treatment and the medical expertise given during these 3 years means that I am now able to work as a dancer, dance artist, teacher and support the development of inclusive dance and practice in the UK and in Sweden. I still have a long way to go to get as well as I want to be, but I am in a very good position and I am definitely on the right track to reach the maximum potential within my own body. I might never do some of the things I thought I would be doing, but without what I have been through I would never have been doing the incredible things that are now part of my life.

Bilateral Total Hip Replacement in a Dancer

Introduction

A case report of a professional contemporary dancer who successfully returned to the stage after bilateral total hip replacements for osteoarthritis is presented, together with a brief retrospective review of hip replacement in dancers.

Case History

T.O, who was born in 1973, started dancing in her native Finland at the age of 7. She later moved to the Rambert School in the UK to complete her training in Contemporary Dance. She then danced professionally with various companies for some 15 years considering herself to have a very slight difference in leg length and a difference in turn-out of about 5 % between the two sides.

She had previously had keyhole surgery on the left knee at the age of 14 though the reason for this was not clear. At the age of 19 surgery was performed to shorten the ligaments at the ankle as an aid to dancing. There was no relevant family history of musculoskeletal disease though her father, who was sporty, had his first hip replacement at the age of 80.

In 2006, at the age of 33 she first noticed pain in the left hip. Initially she attributed this to two particularly complicated pieces of choreography, in one of which she was required to walk on stilts. She considered that the other one might also have placed unilateral strain on the left hip because of the need for high elevations of the right leg. Arthroscopic surgery was performed in 2007 to chisel away a bony spur at the left hip. At this operation the severity of the osteoarthritis in that joint was first realized and a labral tear was also repaired. Figure 7.3 shows an X-ray of both hips at

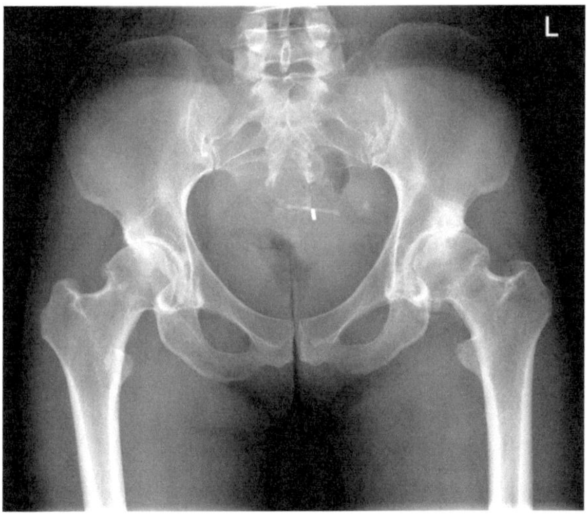

FIGURE 7.3 Pelvic X-ray to show hips, showing severe osteoarthritis on the left side and mild osteoarthritis on the right side. In both cases the degenerative change is relatively localised on the lateral side of the joint

this stage, illustrating that the osteoarthritis particularly affected the lateral part of both hip joints.

Increasingly the range of movement became restricted at the left hip and pain there became more persistent. Plies became more difficult and by 2008 symptoms also commenced in the right hip.

When first reviewed at a Performing Arts Medicine clinic in July 2010 both hips were painful and she demonstrated marked bilateral reduction of internal rotation in flexion at the hips. There was a stiff segment at the base of the spine but the knees, ankles and hips appeared normal. Her general practitioner had already raised the possibility of further hip surgery and she was now referred to an orthopaedic hip specialist. Total left hip replacement was offered and after some consideration she accepted this.

The left hip was therefore replaced with a large bearing ceramic on ceramic prosthesis in September 2010, considered by the surgeon concerned to be the prosthesis most likely to allow her to remain active. Although there was perhaps a paucity of evidence from controlled trials for this relatively new type of prosthesis, the surgeon had previously had good results with it in other sporting groups, especially skiers. He was also very familiar with its use and considered that the large surface areas reduced the risk of future dislocation in a dancer who might still need a wide range of movement at the hip. She was warned of the possible future need for a right total hip replacement and continued with intensive specialized rehabilitation.

No longer dancing on the stage, although the left hip was now largely symptom free, the right hip was becoming increasingly painful and restrictive in terms of her teaching capacity. A large bearing ceramic on ceramic total hip replacement was now offered on the right side and after some deliberation she accepted this as well. The second hip was replaced 1 year after the first (Fig. 7.4).

Rehabilitation could now commence in earnest and she has since returned to full time teaching and demonstrating and in February 2012 returned to the stage for the first time.

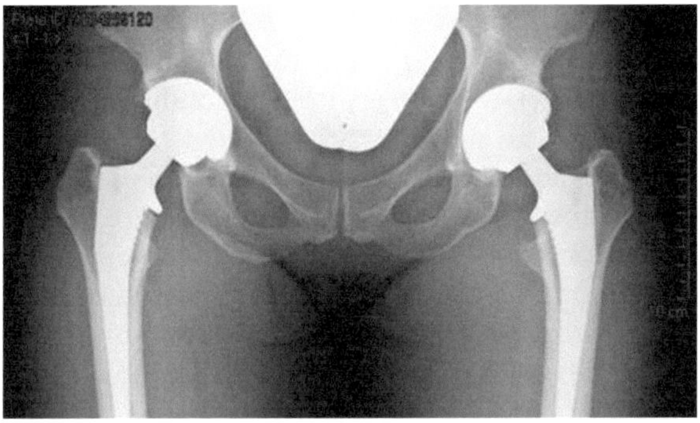

FIGURE 7.4 Post-operative X-ray showing bilateral hip replacements

Interestingly she considers that function is slightly better at the left hip than at the right hip which accords with the X-ray finding that the placement is slightly better positioned on the left side than on the right.

The Patients Viewpoint

Prior to the onset of symptoms I had danced with the Phoenix Dance Theatre in Leeds UK, a company famous for their dancer's athleticism and physical power. I had also enjoyed all forms of movement with activities such as Yoga and Pilates in my spare time. It was difficult to understand what was causing the pain when it first appeared. I had no previous experience in dealing with injury and it became increasingly difficult to lift my left leg to the side. I tried osteopathy, cranial osteopathy, Rolfing and Feldenkrais with varying degrees of success. When things suddenly got worse in the left hip around 2009, I had left the company and was teaching full time though found it increasingly hard to demonstrate and my leg would often give way when I was dancing. It was especially hard to understand why this should have been happening to me.

It has taken a full 2 years for the left hip to regain its many complex functions required for dance although throughout that period I have been pain free. My right side is also now getting stronger, also pain free. By the standards of conventional physiotherapy and function in non-dancers, I was probably back to normal within 3 months of each operation. But that does not take into account the complex and intricate demands dancers make on their bodies. Turn-out, leg lifts and twisting all proved especially hard to regain.

Turn-out positions are still easier to achieve with the left rather than with the right leg, especially when it is raised, but my surgeon suspects this is due to the slightly different position of the two prosthetic sockets. My life is now much happier. It was a challenge to return to a stage performance earlier this year and I really enjoyed the challenge. It provided an opportunity to prove to myself that I had overcome the problem and that I had not been beaten by it.

Although I may never quite have my previous elevation it is lovely to be able to jump and to walk as much as I want without any pain, even though I can still not quite do the splits. My return to the stage was in a work that required considerable physical and emotional effort but which did not require high elevations or difficult lines.

Discussion

In one previous study no significant differences were found in the degenerative changes in the hip joints between former professional female dancers and pair matched controls [1]. Hip complaints are, however, common (21 %; 14/66) in dancers of more than 45 years of age. Forty-three percent of these hip problems were due to degenerative changes in the hip joints [2]. Of this group only three had had a total hip replacement.

It comes as no surprise that the number of total hip replacements in active dancers and dance-teachers is relatively low, even in specialist clinics. In a review of 69 retired dancers, hip and knee complaints were more common than in matched controls though they reported being more content with their lives and experienced being healthier than the controls [3]. No THP replacements were reported in this series.

When surgery is contemplated there are often issues with post-operative expectations which need to be handled sensitively with the dancers concerned. It should always be pointed out that rehabilitation may take as much as a year or even more, much longer than in the general population.

The author has also noted a tendency for some surgeons to offer advice that just concentrates on the affected joint alone. The state of other related joints, in this case the other hip, knees and spine, always needs to be taken in to account before operation is offered.

References

1. van Dijk CN, et al. Degenerative joint disease in female ballet dancers. Am J Sports Med. 1995;23:295–300.
2. Rietveld ABM. Dance injuries in the older dancer: comparison with younger dancers. J Dance Med Sci. 2000;4(1):16–9. 3.
3. Rönnkö R, Heliövaara M, Maimivaara A, Roine R, Seitsalo S, Sainio P, Ketunen J. Musculoskeletal pain, disability and quality of life among retired dancers. J Dance Med Sci. 2007;11(4): 105–9.

Chapter 8
Overuse Syndromes

Introduction

Elite musicians may practise at and play their instrument for some 8 h a day, year in, year out. By athletic standards, this would be anticipated to place strain on those parts of the musculoskeletal system used, in the case of musicians mainly in the arms. Moreover, whilst instruments come in standard pre-determined size; musicians are of varying shape and size. It follows that even with adequate training in technique and sometimes the use of ergonomic aids attached to the instrument, exceptional strain can be placed on instrumentalists who are not suited to their instrument anatomically, compared to those that are. Overuse injury is accepted in sport [1] and 'the over-training syndrome' [2] has been intermittently fashionable. It would stretch credibility if musicians were not to be susceptible to such problems.

Most musicians are extremely dedicated. Their profession is their art such that they have every incentive to remain fit and playing, not least because the profession tends to be over-subscribed. Musicians therefore provide an excellent model for the study of ailments of the arms, once conventional clinical diagnoses have been excluded, since there is often little prospect of successful litigation compared to certain other occupations supported by stronger trade unions. Moreover, musicians are acutely sensitive to the precise onset

H.A. Bird, *Performing Arts Medicine in Clinical Practice*,
DOI 10.1007/978-3-319-12427-8_8,

and localisation of symptoms that have not previously occurred [3], making the profession an excellent model for the study of conditions contentiously termed 'repetitive strain injury' (RSI). Music played prior to or at the onset of symptoms can be analysed in terms of the number of notes required, often allowing surprisingly precise correlation between quite short and specific passages of music and the onset of symptoms. Since choreography is usually also recorded, similar arguments apply to dancers, especially when the choreography is not especially suited to a particular dancer or, more frequently, when the cast for which the piece was designed leaves to be replaced by new dancers of different physique.

This article discusses the current rather unsatisfactory definition of RSI, reviews previous experience of this condition, notably the epidemic that occurred in Australia [4], and highlights particular instrumental pitfalls that may predispose to overuse with certain instruments. It argues, at least on the evidence from musicians, that the syndrome exists but that it is probably not a single entity with a multifactorial aetiology. Accepted medical conditions that may mimic RSI, which probably account for a proportion of all cases, are reviewed with conjecture on the possible overlap with some types of dystonia, a condition covered in a separate article and for which accepted medical guidelines exist.

Work-Related Upper Limb Disorder

For many work-related upper limb disorder (WRULD) has replaced RSI, a term highly suggestive of causation and repetitive strain disorder (RSD), which tended to be confused with the abbreviation for reflex sympathetic dystrophy although it will later be argued that there may be occasional overlap between these two conditions.

The term WRULD tends to be used in the face of persistent symptoms once more conventional medical conditions of the forearm such as tenosynovitis, carpal tunnel syndrome and epicondylitis at the elbow as well as causes of referred pain such as cervical spondylosis have been excluded. It is therfore essentially a diagnosis of exclusion. To suggest it is a function of the industrial age is incorrect. Before the industrial revolution it was endemic in agricultural workers, such as fish workers who, prior to the advent of refrigeration, had to work fast and intermittently as each catch was filleted before it decayed [5]. Clerk's palsy, described 275 years ago, may have been the white collar equivalent even though epidemics of 'writer's cramp' in the British Civil Service around the 1830s were attributed to the introduction of the steel nib [5].

Various aetiologies have been suggested. Amongst these is controlled evidence for certain histological abnormalities in affected patients [6], though others sought to explain the condition in terms of problems with pain amplification [7]. In the case of the Australian epidemic [8], the cumulative growth of symptoms coincided with the introduction of a work compensation system that allowed lump sum payments for work-related disease [9]. Even amongst musicians the unusual frequency of symptoms has been recorded intermittently by many authors over the last 100 years since Poore's first description in 1887 [10, 11].

Various attempts have been made at defining diagnostic criteria [12, 13, Hussain K, 2003, Diagnostic criteria for work related upper limb disorder, personal communication] but none have found universal acceptance.

Problems Specific to Musicians

These are often only highlighted through a meticulous history of playing and performance, sometimes beyond the scope of the doctor lacking experience in this area who may not be familiar with the common instruments and their many variations.

Overuse injury has been defined as 'the damage that occurs when a tissue is stressed beyond its anatomic or physiologic limits, either acutely or chronically' [14]. Some allow this to overlap with tenosynovitis [15], others with damage in the muscle, ligaments and joint capsule [16]. Pathological studies and biopsy studies obviously create ethical difficulties in practising musicians though these have been performed on keyboard operators [17]. The majority of injuries are precipitated by playing [18], particularly an increase in the time and intensity of playing [19].

The piano writing of composer/pianists, always keen to outshine competitors, reflects the unique features of their respective hands. Brahms, Liszt and Rachmaninov all had large hands, Rachmaninov's middle fingers capable of significant lateral movement. By contrast, the piano works of Bach, Mozart and Schumann require a more compact hand. It is the clinical experience of this author that quite short passages of exceptional difficulty can tip the balance into overuse when the player is close to this threshold. If the particular passage is re-fingered, re-structured or even re-composed, the problem is sometimes alleviated.

There are also certain pitfalls among instruments. The commonest is when a violin player transfers to the viola or vice versa. The difference in size and weight of these two instruments creates additional strains to which the performer is unaccustomed. A similar relationship exists between the oboe and cor anglais, the latter instrument being slightly larger and heavier, though mainly with the same fingering. The wide variation between the size and shape of the many members of the saxophone family and the strain that transfer from one of these instruments to another can cause is not always appreciated by the clinician. Although the clarinet and alto saxophone have similar size and fingering, the angle at which the instrument is held is quite different (the saxophone requiring a slight rotation of the spine) and can predispose to overuse, especially if there is a slight natural corkscrew twist of the spine in the opposite direction to that in which the instrument is held.. Spinal scoliosis or rotational twists also causes a problem with the cello since the spine is slightly rotated with the pelvis additionally fixed against the instrument. Although the double bass is a larger more cumbersome instrument, the player has more freedom of spinal movement so this is less likely to occur.

Whilst there is some dispute about the prevalence of thoracic outlet syndrome in musicians, especially amongst violin and viola players [19, 20], the evidence for ulnar nerve entrapment at the elbow whilst playing the violin is much stronger [21] and is normally supported by abnormal nerve conduction studies and EMG. The pressure is thereby localised to the aponeurosis of flexor carpi ulnaris or its underlying fascia.

The complete assessment of musicians requires the musician to be observed playing their instrument. Sometimes the idiosyncrasies of positioning and holding, given the wide diversity of size and shape amongst individuals, clearly demonstrate the compression of soft tissue against a hard surface of the instrument for long periods of time, presenting a risk that is immediately apparent to the physician.

In the experience of this author, the classical guitar and flute are instruments presenting particular problems and account for many referrals to music clinics, once correction is made for the frequency with which these instruments are played. With the classical guitar, significant lateral stretch of the fingers is required in just one hand. Although the flute appears light and easy to play, the position in which it is held is most unergonomic compared to other woodwind instruments, often requiring contortions of the arms and shoulders to accommodate it.

Similar arguments apply to embouchure in brass players and the larynx as an articulation in singers but both are beyond the scope of this review.

Diagnoses that May, in Part, Mimic WRULD

It remains a possibility that if several discreet medical diagnoses are present in the same arm, as can often occur with the complex use of the arm required by musicians, symptoms of each may overlap causing diagnostic confusion. Normally this can be unravelled by a detailed history and careful examination but if a nerve root compression, often at the neck, compounds with a peripheral nerve entrapment, giving an unusual distribution of nerve compression symptoms, this may in part account for the paraesthesiae that are so often a feature of WRULD in musicians.

It is also possible that discreet accepted medical diagnoses, present in mild form, sometimes sub-clinical in respect of clinical examination, may also summate to give symptoms attributable to a WRULD. Eight such possibilities are listed in Table 8.1.

Overuse, as experienced by athletes, is an accepted part of sports medicine [22]. Accepted extrinsic factors felt to contribute include excessive load on the body (both the type and speed of movement and the number of repetitions), training errors (too fast a progression and too high an intensity) and poor equipment. All of this equates with musical training, the instrument representing the equipment.

That micro trauma may be present is partly conjectural but strongly believed by some [17], though this argument is hard to take further in the absence of pathological biopsy material

Table 8.1 Factors that may contribute to symptoms arttributable to "work related upper limb disorder"

1. Overuse (fashionable in athletes)
2. Micro trauma
3. Physiological overload (lactic acidosis)
4. Inherited abnormalities of muscle metabolism
5. Nerve entrapment
6. Compartment syndrome
7. Symptoms are often rare in the self-employed
8. Symptoms may be extremely localised in musicians (perhaps with overlap with focal dystonia as a cortical phenomenon)

from controlled studies, which is largely unethical in professional musicians.

Excessive training, to the point of fatigue and even exhaustion, may invoke physiological results such as lactic acidosis. Lactate accumulates in muscle during exercise [23] and muscle strength, fibre type and enzyme activity all contribute to the severity of this in a given individual [24, 25]. It remains probable that this sort of inter-subject variation occurs in musicians as well as in athletes.

Inherited abnormalities of muscle metabolism such as McArdle's syndrome may also exist in sub-clinical forms, perhaps with partial penetration, which may aggravate the susceptibility to overuse syndrome caused through lactic acidosis.

Peripheral nerve entrapment in violinists is already described above [21]. It has also been described in flautists where the contorted position of the elbow probably predisposes to pressure entrapment [26], certain myelinated conducting fibres probably more susceptible than others [27]. Nerve compression can also occur around the shoulders in musicians [28] where the contour of the cervical and thoracic spines may also contribute.

Compartment syndrome might also be the cause of some symptoms. Here a physical overuse of muscle, restricted within its collagenous fascial sheath produces an increase in pressure which is symptomatic and in severe cases can lead to muscle necrosis. Usually associated with the legs ('shin splints' in dancers), it seems inconceivable that musicians should not be susceptible to this in the arms. Investigation is by the measure of pressure in the muscle compartment and treatment is by surgical release [29]. By implication, both physiological and anatomical features predispose. Examples occur in the arm after surgical trauma [30–32] and it seems feasible that compression of the arm against the firm surface of an instrument might precipitate this as well.

Although unlikely in musicians, it remains a strong possibility that certain psychological factors contribute, especially when symptoms of overuse become established. Thus, overuse syndromes are sometimes felt to be less frequent in the self-employed though this may be artefactual if the self-employed simply adapt a higher threshold for pain in order to continue, working through the symptoms they experience from a genuinely induced pathology.

The precise localisation of symptoms in some musicians is probably attributable entirely to ergonomic factors associated with their specific instrument or, perhaps, the amount of repetitive trauma placed upon a single digit by a particular composition or even a short passage within that composition. Nevertheless, the potential putative overlap with focal dystonia [33] is clear and such dystonias, usually presenting initially in the form of cramps, have been recognised to afflict musicians for some 150 years [34]. Symptoms are often extremely task specific and highly localised in relation to that task. Electromyography often reveals certain abnormalities [35, 36] and the affliction of several elite pianists is undoubted [37].

Aggravating Factors

There is a strong suspicion that certain factors aggravate. One is scoliosis of the spine, particularly with a stringed instruments where a quite different function is required from each of the two arms. Symptoms of this sort are invariably unilateral contrary to a true overuse injury in a keyboard or woodwind player where the symptoms are normally equal and bilateral. In general, this also applies to brass instruments with the exception of the trombone.

There is also a strong clinical impression that joint hypermobility predisposes to overuse syndromes. This would seem logical. Simplistically, extra effort is required to stabilise the hypermobile joint in a position of function before additional effort is applied to move it. In the non-hypermobile joint, the strength of the collagen through the joint capsule and the ligaments, stabilises the joint at rest prior to movement.

Overuse in Dance

It seems probably that most of the above arguments also apply to dancers though here in respect of all parts of the musculoskeletal system, especially the legs and trunk. The muscles and joints concerned are likely to be larger than those in the arm, and invariably will be weight bearing but exactly the same principles apply.

This is partly born out by the acceptance of overuse syndromes or over training syndromes in sport and athletics, for which detailed accounts are available elsewhere.

References

1. Sperryn PN. Overuse injury in sport. Br Med J. 1994;308: 1430–2.
2. Budgett R. The over-training syndrome. Br Med J. 1994;309: 465–8.
3. Charness ME. Unique upper extremity disorders of musicians. In: Millender LH, Louis DS, Simmons BP, editors. Occupational disorders of the upper extremity. New York: Churchill Livingstone; 1992. p. 227–52.
4. Ireland DCR. The Australian experience with cumulative trauma disorders. In: Millender LH, Louis DS, Simmons BP, editors. Occupational disorders of the upper extremity. New York: Churchill Livingstone; 1992. p. 79–88.
5. Great Britain and Ireland Post Office. Departmental Committee on Telegraphists cramp report. London: HMSO; 1911.
6. Dennett X, Fry HJH. Overuse syndrome: a muscle biopsy study. Lancet. 1988;331:905–8.
7. Kellgren JH. Observations on referred pain arising from muscle. Clin Sci. 1938;3:175–90.
8. Hocking B. Epidemiological aspects of 'repetitive strain injury' in Telecom Australia. Med J Aust. 1987;147:218–22.
9. English C, Bird HA. Rheumatological disorders. In: Cox RAF, Edwards FC, Palmer K, editors. Fitness for work: the medical aspects. 3rd ed. Oxford: Oxford University Press; 2000. p. 274–88.

10. Fry HJH. Overuse syndrome in musicians – 100 years ago, an historical review. Med J Aust. 1986;145:620–5.
11. Poore GV. Clinical lecture on certain conditions of the hand and arm which interfere with the performance of professional acts, especially piano playing. Br Med J. 1887;1:441–4.
12. Bird HA, Hill J. Repetitive strain disorder: towards diagnostic criteria. Ann Rheum Dis. 1992;51:974–7.
13. Harrington JM, Carter JT, Birrell L, Gompertz D. Surveillance case definitions for work related upper limb pain syndromes. Occup Environ Med. 1998;55:264–71.
14. Lederman RJ, Calabrese LH. Overuse syndromes in instrumentalists. Med Probl Perform Art. 1986;1:7–11.
15. Newmark J, Hochberg FH. "Doctor, it hurts when I play": painful disorders among instrumental musicians. Med Probl Perform Art. 1987;2:93–8.
16. Fry HJH. Overuse syndrome in musicians. Prevention and management. Lancet. 1986;328:728–31.
17. Dennett X, Fry HJH. Overuse syndrome: a muscle biopsy study. Lancet. 1988;1:905–8.
18. Knishkowy B, Lederman RJ. Instrumental musicians with upper extremity disorders: a follow-up study. Med Probl Perform Art. 1986;1:85–9.
19. Lederman RJ. Thoracic outlet syndromes. Review of the controversies and a report of 17 instrumental musicians. Med Probl Perform Art. 1987;2:87–92.
20. Gilliat RW, Le Quesne PM, Logue V, Sumner AJ. Wasting of the hand associated with a cervical rib or band. J Neurol Neurosurg Psychiatry. 1970;33:615–24.
21. Charness ME, Barbaro NM, Olney RK, Parry GJ. Occupational cubital tunnel syndrome in instrumental musicians. Neurology. 1987;37(3 suppl 1):115.
22. Renstrom PAFH. An introduction to chronic overuse injuries. In: Harries M, Williams C, Stanish WD, Micheli LJ, editors. Oxford textbook of sports medicine. Oxford: Oxford University Press; 1994. p. 531–6.
23. Sjodin B, Svedhenhag J. Assessment of endurance capacity. In: Harries M, Williams C, Stanish WD, Micheli LJ, editors. Oxford textbook of sports medicine. Oxford: Oxford University Press; 1994. p. 172–9.
24. Ivy JL, Withers RT, Van Handel PJ, Elger DH, Costill DL. Muscle respiratory capacity and fiber type as determinants of the lactate threshold. J Appl Physiol. 1980;48:523–7.

25. Essén B, Jansson E, Henriksson J, Taylor AW, Saltin B. Metabolic characteristics of fibre types in human skeletal muscle. Acta Physiol Scand. 1975;95:153–65.
26. Wainapel SF, Cole JL. The not-so-magic flute: two cases of distal ulnar nerve entrapment. Med Probl Perform Art. 1988;3:63–5.
27. Shefner JM, Buchthal F, Krarup C. Slowly conducting myelinated fibers in peripheral neuropathy. Muscle Nerve. 1991;14:534–42.
28. Swift TR, Nichols FT. The droopy shoulder syndrome. Neurology. 1984;34:212–5.
29. Vincent NE. Compartment syndromes. In: Harries M, Williams C, Stanish WD, Micheli LJ, editors. Oxford textbook of sports medicine. Oxford: Oxford University Press; 1994. p. 564–8.
30. Goldie BS, Jones NF, Jupiter JB. Recurrent compartment syndrome and Volkmann contracture associated with chronic osteomyelitis of the ulnar. J Bone Jointt Surg Am. 1990;72:131–3.
31. Hastings H, Misamore G. Compartment syndrome resulting from intravenous regional anaesthesia. J Hand Surg. 1987;12:559–62.
32. Shall J, Cohn BT, Froimson AI. Acute compartment syndrome of the forearm in association with fracture at the distal end of the radius. Report of two cases. J Bone Joint Surg Am. 1986;68:1451–4.
33. Marsden CD, Sheehy MP. Writer's cramp. Trends Neurosci. 1990;13:148–53.
34. Lederman RJ. Neurological problems of performing arts. In: Satalogg RT, Brandfonbrener AG, Lederman RJ, editors. Textbook of performing arts medicine. New York: Raven; 1991. p. 171.
35. Cohen LG, Hallet M. Hand cramps: clinical features and electromyographic patterns in a focal dystonia. Neurology. 1988;38:1005.
36. Hughes M, McLellan DL. Increased co-activation of the upper limb muscles in writer's cramp. J Neurol Neurosurg Psychiatry. 1985;48:782–7.
37. Graffman G. Doctor, can you lend an ear? Med Probl Perform Art. 1986;1:3–6.

Chapter 9
Hypermobility in Dance; Asset Not Liability?

Introduction

Hypermobility, better termed joint laxity, is common in dancers. It has attracted attention ever since Grahame's seminal 1972 paper [1]. There it was argued then that although joint laxity "probably represents the upper end of a spectrum of the range of normal joint mobility," joint hypermobility "may" have positive advantages for ballet dancers, but may also be associated with "its known adverse sequelae". Since then, further papers have published sometimes bleak sounding conclusions that further support this impression.

A key paper from the Royal Ballet in the United Kingdom explored this topic in relation to Joint Hypermobility Syndrome (JHS), pointing to an increased risk of joint symptoms and injury [2] though an accompanying editorial [3] was more circumspect, suggesting some of this may have been partly artifact as a result of problems in study design. The Dutch also are leaders in dance research. A recent paper from Amsterdam [4] cites professional hypermobile dancers to have lower levels of physical fitness, higher levels of fatigue and higher levels of psychological stress (including anxiety and depression) when compared to their non-hypermobile colleagues.

Dancers, who not only encounter such information from university departments of dance science but also from

H.A. Bird, *Performing Arts Medicine in Clinical Practice*, DOI 10.1007/978-3-319-12427-8_9, popular dance magazine and blogs, are often left bemused. Moira McCormack, Head of Physiotherapy for the Royal Ballet Company in London writes that hypermobile students are habitually selected during auditions for vocational dance schools because they are perceived as being "full of potential" [5]. As students progress then, they must work through mixed messages with the moral and psychological complexity of deciding between what is aesthetically pleasing and what is safe –and ultimately, what will secure their income. Hypermobile dancers are left to worry whether they might be "accidents waiting to happen" or worse, whether their lifetime of intensive training was for nothing because their body structures are genetically pre-determined to physically fall short of their ultimate career placements.

Problems with the Scoring Systems

Many dancers rely on the existing scoring systems for joint hypermobility. These established scoring systems that have been developed and utilized by doctors for assessment of their patients are invariably used when studies are conducted on dancers. This is unfortunate because from the perspectives of the dancer participants, the scoring systems only consider a small number of joints and do not consider all the various arcs of movement in which they can move and bend their bodies.

The Beighton scoring system of 1973 [6] is described and illustrated in Table 9.1 and Fig. 9.1 respectively. This, initially adapted from earlier 1964 criteria by Carter and Wilkinson [7] was devised for use in large-scale epidemiological studies in a rural South African population where a rapid 30-s assessment of each individual was all that was required. By contrast, the Brighton Criteria, published in 2000 [8] and listed in Table 9.2, were devised mainly for the evaluation of patients who displayed extra-articular and painful symptoms in clinics. Crucially neither criteria set was designed specifically for use in the dance population.

TABLE 9.1 The 9 point Beighton scoring system for measuring joint hypermobility

One point is scored on each side for the following
Passive dorsiflexion of the 5th metacarpo-phalangeal joint to 90°
Apposition of the thumb to the flexor aspect of the forearm
Hyperextension of the elbow beyond 0°
Hyperextension of the knee beyond 0°
One point is scored for
Forward flexion of the trunk so the hands are placed flat on the floor with the knees extended
Maximum score: 9 points
(These positions are shown in diagrammatic form in Fig. 9.1)

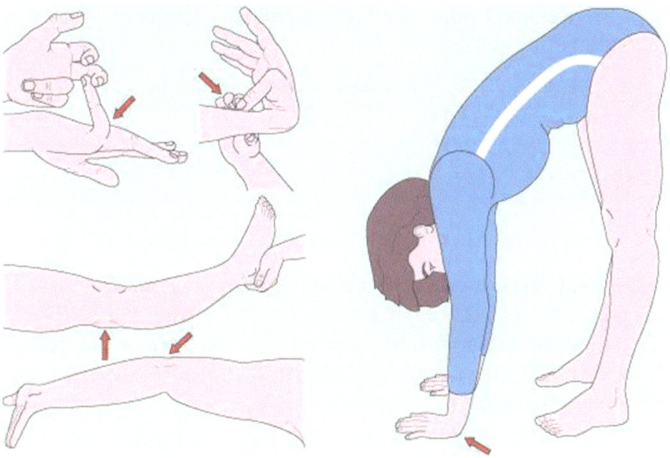

FIGURE 9.1 Beighton (1973) criteria in diagrammatic form (With permission from Elsevier Hochberg et al. [25])

Even within rheumatology, opinion differs on the value of such criteria. The British Society for Rheumatology recently

TABLE 9.2 The Brighton criteria for joint hypermobility syndrome

Major criteria
A Beighton score of 4/9 or more, either currently or historically
Arthralgia for longer than 3 months in four or more joints
Minor criteria
A Beighton score of 1, 2 or 3/9 (or 0, 1, 2 or 3 if aged greater than 50)
Arthralgia (<3 months) in one to three joints or back pain (<3 months), spondylosis, spondylolysis, spondylolisthesis
Dislocation/subluxation in more than one joint or in one joint on more than one occasion
Soft tissue rheumatism >3 lesions (e.g. epicondylitis, tenosynovitis, bursitis)
Marfanoid habitus: tall, slim, span/height ratio >1.03, upper/lower segment ratio <0.89, arachnodactyly (positive Steinberg/wrist signs)
Abnormal skin: striae, hyperextensibility, thin skin, papyraceous scarring
Eye signs; drooping eyelids or myopia or anti-mongoloid slant
Varicose veins or hernia or uterine/rectal prolapse
The Joint Hypermobility Syndrome (JHS) is diagnosed in the presence of TWO major criteria, or ONE major and TWO minor criteria, or FOUR minor criteria. Two minor criteria will suffice where there is an unequivocally affected first degree relative.
Criteria Major 1 and Minor 1 are mutually exclusive as are Major 2 and Minor 2.
JHS is excluded by the presence of Marfan or Ehlers-Danlos Syndromes (other than the EDS hypermobility type; formerly EDS type 3) as defined by the [26] and the [27] criteria respectively.

sponsored an interactive debate. As co-chair, one of us (HB) felt surprised that 76 % of the audience were still using the Beighton criteria but was less surprised that only 21 % were using the Brighton criteria. The Brighton criteria tend to attract criticism in that when major criterion number 2 is paired with minor criterion number 4, a combination that might be found in many patients visiting any rheumatology clinic, considerable trust is placed in the discriminatory power of the single further minor criterion needed to clinch the diagnosis of HMS.

Additional problems arise when applying objective, medical scores to the dynamic movement capabilities of dancers. For example, range of motion in the hips when muscles and connective tissues are warm can change significantly when compared to measurements taken 'cold' or when dancers feel fatigued. Moreover, the specific ways one stretches the body in order to measure it, need to be considered. Dynamic stretching -when the body moves via muscle contraction- is much different to static stretching, when the movement is achieved through external force [9]. Sometimes, the difference in flexibility between these two types of stretching is substantial. These factors need to become consistent features of research methodology.

In addition, recording of injuries by interview or questionnaire tends not to account for the magnitude of the force causing the injury, which, in the case of dance may be substantial. There is even some evidence that in the case of the most serious injuries, hypermobility with its inherent properties of shock absorbency may act as a protecting factor.

There is now an urgent need for new scoring systems devised and validated in dancers to complement methods already established in the evaluation of other aspects of their performance. One example of such a development is Redding's dance aerobic fitness test (DAFT) for the evaluation of dance capabilities at low to moderate levels of intensity [10]. The additional *high intensity fitness test* measures both a dancer's aerobic and anaerobic systems— a condition more specific to performance demands [11, 12]. These tests are conducted in a studio so dancers can comfortably perform to the best of their ability using different muscle groups at different times with varying levels of impact. Furthermore, qualitative methods such as the recording of subjective visual observations and subsequent analysis of the participants' movements are utilized. These types of adaptations are much more credible and transferable to the complex world of the dance artist. A further promising test for balance has been devised [13] but still awaits full validation.

The Different Causes of Hypermobility

Whatever the value of scoring systems, an appreciation of the several different factors that contribute to the observed range of movement at a given joint informs much more on pathogenesis and management. It is normally accepted that four factors can contribute [14], the proportion of each varying not only between individuals but also from joint to joint in the same individual. The four factors are the shape of the bony articulating surfaces, the structure of the collagen, the functioning of the muscles and the nervous system control of the musculoskeletal system. Some of these are inherited, others acquired or modified through learning and training.

An association between joint laxity and congenital dislocation of the hip was first described in 1964 [7], in a paper that also defined a scoring system that preceded that proposed by Beighton et al. [6]. That a hip joint with a shallow socket, determined genetically, should have a wider range of movement than a hip joint with a deep socket is obvious though any laxity of the collagen in the joint capsule will clearly contribute as well. A very wide variety of skeletal dysplasias [15, 16] contribute to joint laxity through bony structure at a wide variety of sites, many of which are associated subtle skeletal clues [17] such as the shape of the toes, feet or fingers and often with subtle degrees of spinal scoliosis. This type of laxity is unlikely to be influenced significantly by warm-up. Often a small number of joints are disproportionately flexible.

The structure of collagen also varies substantially between individuals, displaying various degrees of elasticity. More detailed descriptions are available elsewhere [18] Clues here are that this is associated with easy bruising, hernia formation, skin elasticity and probably some degree of oversensitivity in the sympathetic nervous system. This type of laxity is spread evenly across many joints across the body and is only modestly increased by warm-up.

Muscles serve to stabilize joints, partly by their bulk but also by their consistency, which is influenced both by the strength of the collagen that makes up the fascia in each muscle but also by the sensitivity of the contractility. This clearly differs simultaneously between agonists and antagonists if movement and balance is to be achieved. Flexibility can therefore be enhanced both by stretching the fascia but also by adjusting the muscle tone. A clue here is the long warm-up that is required though this can increase the range of movement as much as anything.

Finally there has recently been increasing interest in the neurophysiology. Proprioception is known to be impaired in hypermobile joints, possibly because the stretch receptors work inefficiently in a lax joint [19]. There is also thought to be a basic abnormality in the reflex arc (Ferrell WR, 2013, personal communication). Clues to this type of laxity are clumsiness as a child and delayed walking as well as poor spatial awareness though clearly, mechanical factors may contribute to these symptoms as well.

In any one individual, all of these causes will coalesce to varying degree to produce the final observed phenotype. Understanding of the contribution of each determinant informs on the optimum training methods most suitable to each individual and the style of dance to which they aspire (Table 9.3).

TABLE 9.3 Causes of observed hypermobility

Shape of the articulating surfaces (Refs. [7, 15, 16])
Structure of collagen (Ref. [18])
Muscular tone (Refs. [5, 9])
Joint proprioception (Refs. [19, Ferrell WR, 2013, personal communication])
Any or all of these influence the observed range of movement at a given joint

Hormonal Aspects

Epidemiologically, joint laxity varies with age, is more marked in females in most ethnic groups, varies slightly with menstruation and is much more marked during pregnancy, a feature that normally persists throughout breast-feeding. Joint laxity can also become more severe and more painful in the presence of gynaecological conditions such as polycystic ovary and endometriosis. Clearly hormones, especially the female sex hormones contribute, probably through their effect on collagen structure but perhaps also through subtle effects on proprioception. It is thus very common for hyperlax females to notice looseness of the joints associated with clumsiness at the times when the menstrual cycle is progestogen dominated.

This may be regulated by the use of appropriate contraceptives but progesterone only preparations often (though not always) make things worse. A combined oral contraceptive pill is more likely to provide stability and there seems to be some variation between the various preparations according to the structure of the progesterone component. If this is an issue, it may be advisable to try several in turn.

Psychological Aspects

The association between hypermobility and certain psychiatric disorders appears complex, still not fully understood. Certain disorders, for example panic disorder, agoraphobia, and simple phobias are more common in hypermobile patients than controls [20]. Conversely, joint laxity is 16 times more common in persons with panic attacks than in controls [21]. The most convincing evidence comes from a community-based study establishing beyond doubt an association between anxiety (panic) disorder and joint laxity [22]. This probably reflects linkage on the same chromosome [23].

These associations could have implications on dance training. A performer more prone to feeling anxious may need special attention during rehearsals or before performances to relieve stress. Certain action plans or cognitive-behavioural routines could be tailored to fit a dancer's temperament and to aid them in the event of an attack. Also, a dancer might use stretching as a technique to relieve symptoms of anxiety, which has the potential to disturb their already precarious balance of the strength to flexibility ratio. Teachers should maintain attentive to such potentialities, as it could affect a dancer's physical stability and chances of falling victim to injury.

A Strategy for the Future

Individualized support for the hypermobile dancer is ideal. Critchfield, in her 2011 IADMS information sheet [9] states that in respect to flexibility, "dancers should experiment carefully under the direction of experienced teachers or health care professionals to find the optimal stretching technique for their physique."

With specific attention allocated to a dancer, it is possible to pinpoint and manage the factors contributing to their type and level of hypermobility, which may vary in degree throughout the body. Rather than using scoring systems that simply count joints, both dance and medical professionals need to analyze *why* each joint is flexible. With a thorough examination of personal and family history and, if necessary, even X-rays and –MRIs, a 'flexibility profile' could be developed for each dancer and then addressed accordingly.

Based on the dancer's flexibility profile – encompassing both physical and psychological factors – professionals could correlate the development of a conditioning program with the performance requirements of the particular genre of movement to which the dancer aspires. Each dance style demands a unique skill set and most dancers benefit from the ability to adapt to more than one style.

This highly specialized plan, with training procedures and movement exercises that are safely adapted to the dancer's body, does not necessarily need to come from the dance world alone. Sports science research informs on highly effective methods for enhancing endurance, balance, and proprioception. And, depending on the dancer's needs, anatomical localization of strengthening and stretching, either its enhancement or reduction, can be pursued. Through this work, dancers can feel more secure pursuing and maintaining employment.

Certain disciplines, which seem particularly appropriate to dance training such as Pilates, Gyrotonic ®, and Yoga, especially Ashtangar (or Power Yoga) are currently under study.

A recent article in the UK Foundations for Excellence series [24] written by an amateur dancer, the senior physiotherapist at the Royal Ballet, and a physician with over 20 years experience of treating joint laxity in dancers concluded that hypermobility was highly prevalent amongst dancers but that a greater understanding of the many factors that contribute to the condition was required and that "these dancers should be given specialized attention and support during training if injury is to be avoided and their potential fully realized". This remains an important objective in the support and care of all hypermobile dancers.

References

1. Grahame R, Jenkins JM. Joint hypermobility; asset or liability? A study of joint mobility in ballet dancers. Ann Rheum Dis. 1972;39:109–11.
2. McCormack M, Briggs J, Hakim A, Grahame R. Joint laxity and the benign joint hypermobility syndrome in student and professional ballet dancers. J Rheumatol. 2004;31:173–8.

3. Bird HA. Rheumatological aspects of dance. J Rheumatol. 2004;31:12–3.
4. Scheper MC, de Vries JE, de Vos R, Verbunt J, Nollet F, Engelbert RHH. Generalized joint hypermobility in professional dancers; a sign of talent or vulnerability? Rheumatology. 2013;52(4):651–8.
5. McCormack M. Teaching the hypermobile dancer. IADMS Bull Teach. 2010;2(1):1–5.
6. Beighton PH, Solomon L, Soskolne CL. Articular mobility in an African population. Ann Rheum Dis. 1973;32:413–7.
7. Carter C, Wilkinson J. Persistent joint laxity and congenital dislocation of the hip. J Bone Joint Surg Br. 1964;46-B:40–4.
8. Grahame R, Bird HA, Child A, et al. The revised (Brighton 1988) criteria for the diagnosis of benign joint hypermobility syndrome. J Rheumatol. 2000;27:1777–9.
9. Critchfield B. Stretching for dancers. 2011. Published by International Association for Dance Medicine and Science at their website. www.Dancescience.org.
10. Wyon M, Redding E, Abt G, Head A, Sharp C. Development, reliability and validity of a multi-stage dance specific aerobic fitness test (DAFT). J Dance Med Sci. 2003;7(3):80–4.
11. Redding E, Weller P, Ehrenberg S, Irvine S, Quin E, Rafferty S, Wyon M, Cox C. The development of a high intensity dance performance fitness test. J Dance Med Sci. 2009;13:1–8.
12. Redding E. Testing for high intensity dance fitness. IADMS Bull Teach. 2009;1:14–6.
13. Batson G. Validating a dance-specific screening test for balance: Preliminary results from multisite testing. Med Probl Perform Art. 2012;103–8.
14. Joint hypermobility. Patient information sheet published by Arthritis Research UK. 2011. www.arthritisresearchuk.org.
15. International working group on Constitutional Diseases of Bone. International nomenclature and classification of the osteochondrodysplasias (1997). Am J Med Genet. 1998;79(5):376–82.
16. Shapiro F. Pediatric orthopaedic defeormities. Basic science, diagnosis and treatment. San Diego: Academic; 2001.
17. Jones KL. Smith's recognizable patterns of human malformation. 5th ed. London/Philadelphia: WB Saunders; 1997.
18. Kadler K, Wallis G. The molecular basis of joint hypermobility. In: Beighton P, Grahame R, Bird H, editors. Hypermobility of joints. 4th ed. London: Springer; 2012.

19. Ferrell WR, Tennant N, Sturrock RD, et al. Amelioration of symptoms by enhancement of proprioception in patients with joint hypermobility syndrome. Arthritis Rheum. 2004;50:3323–8.
20. Bulbena A, Duro JC, Mateo A, Porta M, Vallejo J. Joint hypermobility syndrome and anxiety disorders. Lancet. 1988;2(8612):694.
21. Bulbena A, Duro JC, Porta M, et al. Anxiety disorders in the joint hypermobility syndrome. Psychiatry Res. 1993;46(1):59–68.
22. Martin-Santos R, Bulbena A, Porta M, Gago J, Molina L, Duro JC. Association between joint hypermobility syndrome and panic disorder. Am J Psychiatry. 1998;155:1579–83.
23. Gratacós M, Nadal M, M-Santos R, et al. A polymorphic genomic duplication on human chromosome 15 is a susceptibility factor for panic and phobic disorders. Cell. 2001;106(3):367–79.
24. Knight I, McCormack M, Bird HA. Managing joint hypermobility; a guide for teachers. 2012. Foundations for Excellence. Published by South West Music School, PO box 730, Exeter EX1 9RA.
25. Hochberg MC, et al. Rheumatology. 3rd ed. Mosby; Edinburgh, London, NY. 2003.
26. Beighton P. International nosology of hereditable disorders of connective tissue, Berlin, 1986. Am J Med Genet. 1988;29: 581–94.
27. Beighton P, De Paepe A, Steinmann B, Tsipouras P, Wenstrup RJ. Ehlers-Danlos syndromes:revised nosology, Villefranche 1997. Am J Med Genet. 1998;77:31–7.

Chapter 10
Scoliosis in Musicians and Dancers

Introduction

Traditionally scoliosis (Ancient Greek; 'bending') is a condition in which the spine is curved from side to side. On x-ray, viewed from the rear, the spine of an individual with scoliosis may be shaped like an 'S' or a 'C' rather than straight. In the performing artist, the classification becomes more complicated. Simplistically, an 'S-shaped' curve is compensated whilst a C-shaped curve is not, requiring the pelvis to be tilted. Sometimes scolioses viewed from front to back are even more complicated, an S adjacent to a C, for example, which would also be uncompensated. Once local disease of the hip is excluded, an uncompensated scoliosis is one of the commonest causes of a slight difference in the leg length.

By definition, a curve viewed from front to back also creates a small degree of corkscrew twist in the spine. Sometimes a corkscrew twist is the predominant feature; the 'S-shaped' curve is secondary to this. Here, according to whether the corkscrew is compensated or uncompensated, there may be a pelvic twist as well as a tilt, exemplified especially in dancers by unequal turnout as well as difference in leg length.

In the context of performing arts, the contour of the spine viewed from the side needs to be considered as well although the hyper-flexion of a kyphosis or the hyperextension of a lordosis is often classified separately. A variety of alternative

H.A. Bird, *Performing Arts Medicine in Clinical Practice*,
DOI 10.1007/978-3-319-12427-8_10,

classifications exist reflecting aetiology, including congenital, idiopathic or neuromuscular. However, for musicians and dancers the anatomical configuration rather than the pathogenesis is usually the most important feature in their management.

Invariably, degrees of scoliosis are associated with a wide variety of minor congenital abnormalities in the spine, not always described in the conventional radiological report. Sometimes this can be extreme as in the case of Chiari malformation; more frequently an unusual shape of a vertebra goes unnoticed, any abnormality argued to be within the variation that could be expected within a normal population.

A scoliosis that may be asymptomatic in a sedentary individual is often rendered symptomatic through participation in the art form. To play an instrument of standard size, irrespective of body shape, contour or height, creates an ergonomic situation not usually found in a normal population, especially if the instrumentalist is practising for around 6 h a day. The scoliosis may also be rendered symptomatic by dance but here the spine is rarely held rigid for long periods. Dance, as an art form, provides ample scope for self-physiotherapy and for the adoption of an individual technique that compensates for any restriction caused by the scoliosis.

When scoliosis is found in a child or adolescent, the lay advice instinctively given is that a career as an instrumentalist would be 'safer' than a career as a dancer. Experience from performing arts clinics suggests that this is not always true.

This article reviews cases of scoliosis seen in three performers, a violinist, a cellist and a dancer. Applied physiotherapy has been invaluable in each case but symptoms in the two string players, where the completely different function required of the two sides of the body often compounds the problem, has arguably been less successful than treatment of the dancer who returned successfully to performing.

Scoliosis in a Violinist

TC was first seen in 2011 at the age of 55. A professional violinist, playing since adolescence, she had a previous history of detached retina on two occasions, cataracts, mild hypertension and early osteoarthritis of the hands. Previously there had been a right Achilles tendinosis.

On New Year's Eve 2010 at around 20.00 h she developed a sudden onset of pain affecting the right shoulder and the right upper arm, occurring as she was dressing for a party. The symptoms were unilateral and so severe that a heart attack was initially suspected. This had never occurred before and there were no clues in the previous history. The next day the husband noticed winging of the right scapula. The pain resolved after 1 week but winging of the scapula persisted. Her violin playing was therefore compromised, especially when she was playing on the G and D strings.

On referral to a consultant rheumatologist the strong clinical impression was that she had a neuritis, probably viral in aetiology, involving the right long thoracic nerve. This was confirmed beyond doubt on nerve conduction studies. She was offered physiotherapy at her local hospital but this failed to remedy the situation.

Subsequent nerve conduction studies, performed when the right scapula was still winged and there was significant weakness of serratus anterior and mild weakness of the rhomboids showed severe partial denervation in the right serratus anterior only, the other muscles spared electro-physiologically. There was some fibrillation and very poor recruitment of muscle units in the right serratus anterior.

In June 2011 she was referred specifically to a clinic of performing arts medicine where her recent x-rays were reviewed in the light of the neuro-physiological findings. The bulk of evidence clearly supported pathology at the serratus anterior through involvement of the long thoracic nerve, now largely resolving spontaneously, but the cause of this remained uncertain. The history was perhaps against a viral neuritis and the onset of symptoms very sudden, almost instantaneous. Review of the x-rays showed significant curving of both the cervical (Figs. 10.1 and 10.2) and thoracic spine raising the possibility that compression of the long thoracic nerve was largely biomechanical.

Physiotherapy subsequently was devoted more to the spine than to the shoulder girdle as before, with consequent improvement.

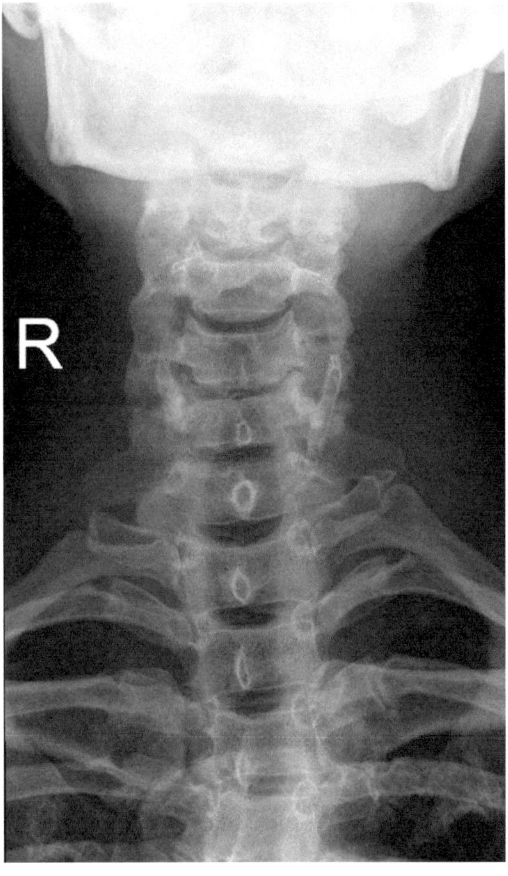

FIGURE 10.1 PA X-ray of neck

Comment

This case illustrates how a longstanding scoliosis of the thoracic spine, probably congenital and previously unnoticed, can cause unexpected neurological symptoms. A compensatory twist in the cervical spine where it was associated with

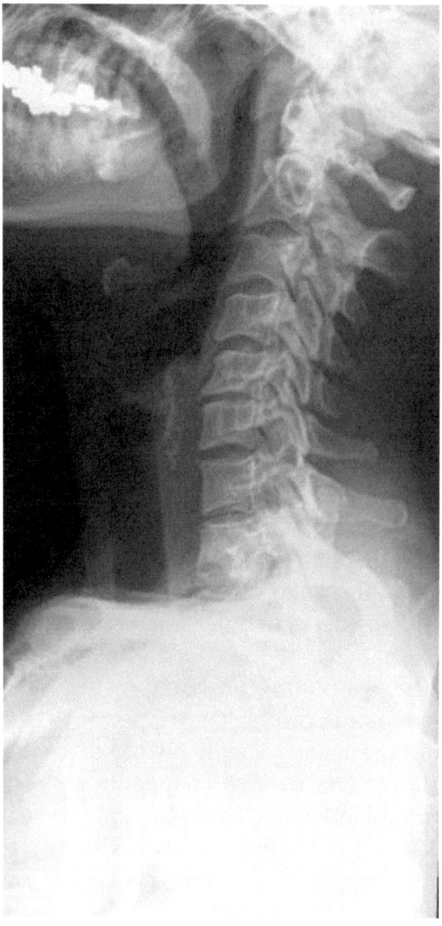

FIGURE 10.2 Lateral X-ray of neck

some degenerative change compounded the problems of violin playing at a professional level. When management was directed towards the spine symptoms improved. It remains probable that playing technique had been compromised gradually over a long period of time, the player instinctively making adaptations to her predicament as often occurs. A sudden event, possibly traumatic in onset, perhaps even as she was dressing into party clothes, precipitated the problem. With applied informed physiotherapy, improvement occurred and she is now back playing, compensating easily through her technique for the progressive mild degenerative changes in the fingers and the cervical spine.

Mild Scoliosis in a Cellist

KA was first seen at a performing arts medicine clinic in March 2006 when she was 25, having sought help over the previous 2 years at other general clinics as well as one devoted to performing arts medicine where her joint hypermobility had been noted.

As a child she was talented at both music and dance, self-driven to have lessons at both and to excel. Her principal instrument was the cello, the piano her second. Her joint hypermobility assisted her talent at ballet and she danced seriously until the age of 13 years and played the cello seriously until the age of 15 years. By now she was developing some joint symptoms, probably attributable to hypermobility, and in view of these and a family history of joint disease (her younger sister was born with congenital dislocation of the hips and her father had severe osteoarthritis of the knee), well-intentioned family advice was to concentrate on music. She also had a painful ganglion at the right wrist. When she tore a ligament there this was corrected surgically, which led to a partial fusion of the right wrist, making it very difficult for her to play. She had also given up her career in dance and was studying for a theoretical musical degree that required some practical performance.

When first seen in March 2006 the main problem was severe debilitating pain in the thoracic spine. This was aggravated by the heavy lifting required in her temporary job, then as a nursing auxiliary in a care home. She also sought career guidance, the cello still her first love.

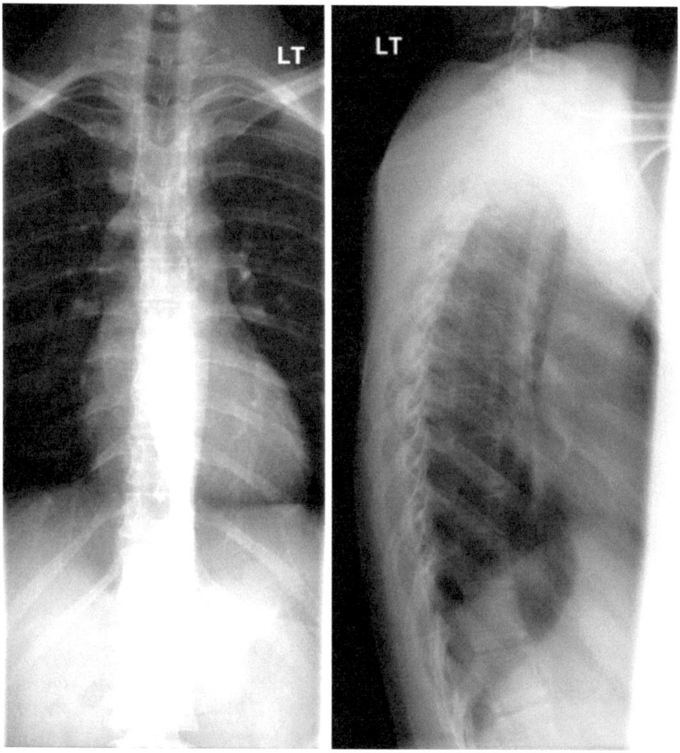

FIGURE 10.3 2006 Plain X-ray of thoracic spine. However an MRI scan performed soon after showed the presence multiple Schmorl's nodes, the largest at T6

On examination, joint hypermobility was extreme, most marked at the shoulder, which subluxed downwards on minimal provocation, compounding the difficulty of playing the cello because of the fused right wrist. The spine was flexible in all arcs of movement, particularly hyperextension. She considered herself the most flexible of the three siblings.

Investigations in March 2006 showed thoracic spine felt to be normal on X-ray (Fig. 10.3) but an MRI confirmed the presence of Schmorl's nodes, by far the largest of these at the level of T6, the site of her pain, which was also the mid-point of a slight intra-thoracic scoliosis with an element of corkscrew twist. This tended to fix the spine largely in the rotational direction opposite to that of the slight rotation required to play the cello.

Management was with painkillers and a combination of extensive active physiotherapy directed at the thoracic spine and the scoliosis with the Schmorl's nodes, with the reintroduction of the exercises required for dance. She found stretching exercises perhaps the most helpful in relieving symptoms, particularly when these mobilised the thoracic spine.

She subsequently proceeded to a career in university administration, continuing to play the cello and piano recreationally and to give lessons in these instruments. She has therefore retained the valuable antique cello she was bequeathed when she showed such promise as a child prior to her operation.

Comment

This case illustrates several points of interest. A very mild scoliosis, often particularly problematic in cellists when there is a corkscrew element in the thoracic spine in the wrong direction, was here complicated by the presence of Schmorl's nodes. A variety of spinal conditions, some hereditary, can occur in conjunction with an inherited scoliosis, which must always be kept in mind as a cause of symptoms. The case illustrates the value of physiotherapy in relieving pain. Dance and stretching exercises proved particularly helpful in her case and one has to speculate that the well-intentioned family and medical advice given when she discontinued her dance to concentrate on her instrument, in retrospect was probably wrong. Career guidance in the adolescent who is talented as a performing artist is crucial especially when, as so often, they are talented in both music and dance.

Scoliosis and Vertebral Abnormalities in a Dancer

ED who only reached a specialist clinic at the age of 23, had always shown talent as a dancer (ballet, tap and modern) since the age of 9 years. She trained for 7 years at her local dance school and, at the age of 17 years, proceeded to a 3-year diploma at a dance college specialising in musical theatre, though she also obtained teaching qualifications. She then worked professionally for 1 year on cruise ships. She had considerable power, average endurance and better than average flexibility as a result of training. A slight difference in leg length had been suspected on several occasions and there was a significant difference in turnout.

Musculoskeletal problems commenced in early 2009 while dancing on the cruise liner, initially pain in one shoulder then a problem with the right hamstring, then problems with the left hip and the right foot.

She consulted a variety of physiotherapists, podiatry doctors and musculoskeletal clinicians before she finally reached a performing arts clinic in April 2010, referred from her local consultant rheumatologist.

The main problem then was lower back pain, though the unilateral preponderance of symptoms at peripheral joints, so typical of spinal imbalance normally through scoliosis, was striking.

On examination the difference in turnout was around 30° in a resting position and the slight difference in leg length was confirmed. One hip joint moved more easily than the other and there was clear asymmetry of muscular mass adjacent to the spine in the thoracic region as well as asymmetry of scapula movement when the arms were raised above the head. At that stage she had not been able to dance for 18 months because of spinal pain, in spite of some 12 years training to become a professional dancer.

X-rays showed several findings expected as a result of clinical examination. Thus, there was no evidence of

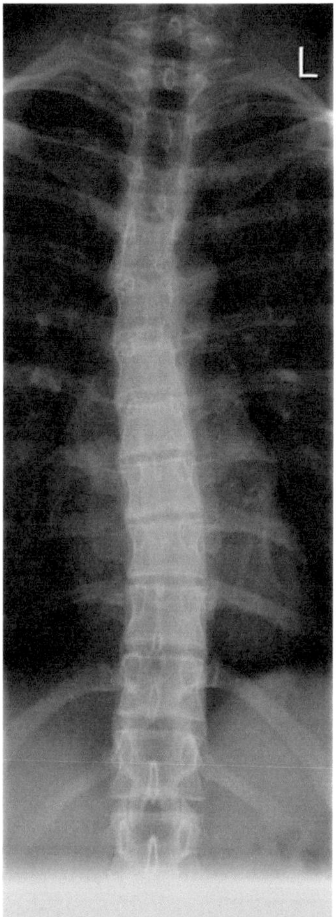

FIGURE 10.4 X-ray of thoracic spine

inflammatory arthritis or degenerative change and the sacroiliac joints were normal. A significant 'S-shaped' scoliosis confined within the thoracic spine, concaved to the left between T1 and T6 and concave to the right between T7 and T12 was confirmed with angulation at the mid-point around T6 (Fig. 10.4). An unexpected finding, not apparent from examination, was of a dysmorphic (transitional) fifth lumbar vertebra, which showed sacrolisation such that the right

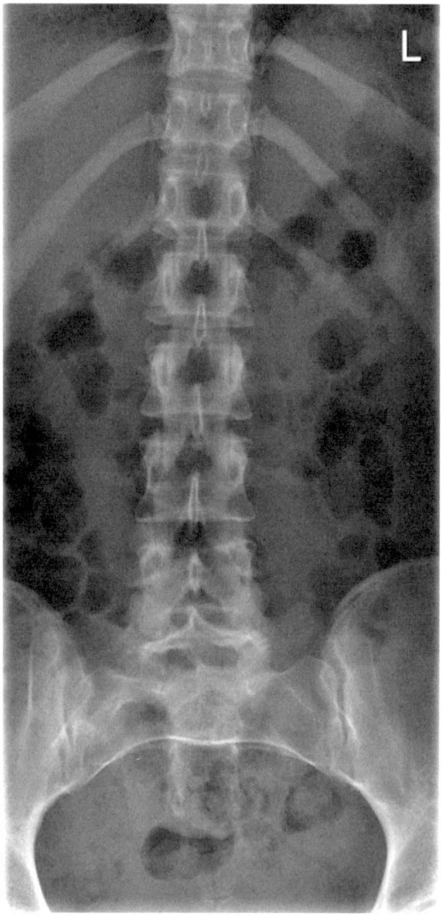

FIGURE 10.5 X-ray of lumbar spine

transverse process only was fused to the pelvis (Figs. 10.5 and 10.6). In turn, this rather than a corkscrew twist higher in the spine was felt to be the cause of the slightly rotated pelvis, explaining the difference in turnout. This, one of the two main sites of her spinal pain (the other being around T6) led to a localised stiff segment, which prevented any compensation for the rigidity of the thoracic scoliosis above it, the clinical importance of which had not previously been

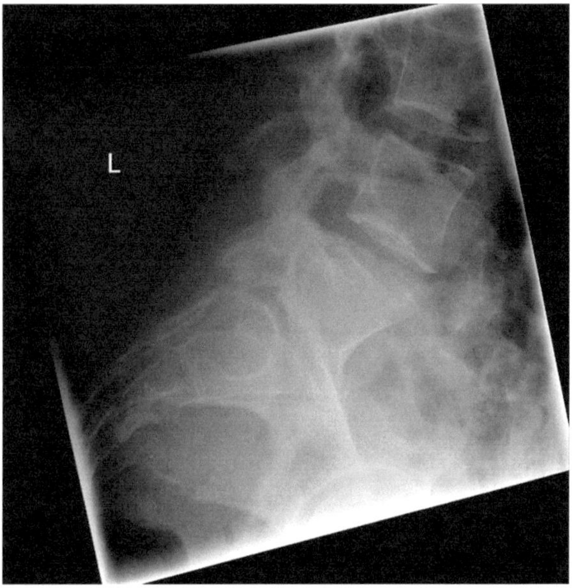

FIGURE 10.6 Transitional vertebra at L5

appreciated by either the dancer or any of her previous many medical attendants.

A strategic decision was made not to attempt to mobilise the L5/S1 region but to strengthen this with appropriate exercises and leave it as a stiff segment. On balance, it was felt that mobilisation of the thoracic spine, the second most stiff segment, would be relatively unrewarding. A physiotherapy programme was therefore devised, which vigorously mobilised the spine between T12 and L4 in compensation for the lack of movement at other levels. Subsequent Pilates and PNF (proprioceptive neuromuscular facilitation) techniques were introduced and this combination of applied treatments, quite different and specific for each of the segments of her spine, allowed her return to dancing professionally in public by June 2011, approximately 1 year after the introduction of specific techniques.

Comment

This case illustrates the importance of accurate diagnosis at all levels of the spine and the complexity of specialist management when compensation is not available at parts of the spine distant from the scoliosis. Once this was appreciated and the spine treated as separate individual segments, symptoms and function improved dramatically leading to a return to dancing in public after 1 year. The skill with which dancers, as opposed to musicians, understand and self-manipulate their joints, especially segments of the spine, together with the active movement and the muscular strengthening, co-ordination and control that dance provides, all bode well for recovery.

A Physiotherapy Perspective

It is uncommon for a performing artist, dancer or musician, to consult a health practitioner about a scoliosis. Usually the individual will have complaints of pain or repetitive injury and, only after examination is the scoliosis is detected. This structural abnormality of the spine most commonly develops in periods of growth spurt like the one that occurs between the age of 5 and 8 years of life, which matches the time when most children start extracurricular activities like dance and music [1]. It is often hard, however, to separate inherited and acquired components [2]. This is especially true in string players where the two sides of the body have quite separate functions when playing music. Here remedial exercises may redress the balance, especially when the abnormality is the result of the posture required in the playing of a stringed instrument.

Scoliosis is often overlooked when is mild and compensated (under 10° of scoliosis the diagnosis of scoliosis should not be made and these less severe curves often remain stable [3]). It tends to be asymptomatic and the patient is free to keep doing their normal activities without restraint. However, when an individual is engaged in a more demanding or extreme physical activity they become susceptible to developing symptoms associated with their pre-existent scoliosis [4]. Despite the common misconception that this is a problem of athletes, performing artists are also very much afflicted. The literature shows that scoliotic patients prefer to practice sports like gymnastics (usually started before discovering the scoliosis) which is also to linked to a higher prevalence of joint laxity [5]. This sort of joint laxity is also highly sought after by both dancers, for the lower limb and musicians, for the upper limb.

Dancers are subjected to intense physical activity that, due to its artistic component, tends to reach extreme limits of anatomy and physiology in an episodic fashion, according to season and employment, which can trigger symptoms in an otherwise asymptomatic scoliosis. Some studies show that, specifically in ballet dancers, the prevalence of scoliosis is increased. The different types of curve found in this population suggest that the exercise pattern may determine which type of scoliosis is developed (but not the curve severity). This finding supports the ideas that scoliotic ballet dancers should be classified in a different category of scoliosis: sports-associated scoliosis [1]. For musicians, the extreme nature of their physical activity lies on the repetitive nature of their practice and performance. Being dedicated to one instrument around 7 h per day fosters the strain, stress and stretch of the same muscles and joints repeatedly.

With the unstable nature of their work and, at many times, a lack of physical support, performers are used to enduring a certain amount of pain and tend to only resort to health practitioners when the symptoms prevent them from playing or dancing. Even within a "normal" population, scoliotic adults suffer from spinal pain, which they experience more frequently than non-scoliotic adults. Statistically significant differences are already found in people between 20 and 30 years of age [3], and this effect is enhanced in performers.

As physiotherapeutic specific exercises (PSE) are recommended as the first step to treat idiopathic scoliosis to prevent/limit progression of the deformity, these same exercises can often be helpful for performers. The frequency of therapeutic sessions depends on the techniques, cooperation and the ability of the patient to carry out the treatment. It is recommended that PSE should be based on auto-correction in 3D, stabilizing of the corrected posture and patient education. Also exercises should be individualized according to patient's needs, activity, work pattern with treatment phased and delivered regularly.

Sports activities have been suggested as an active counterpart of PSE [3] so dancers should be encouraged not to stop practicing when a scoliosis is diagnosed, but rather to shape their practice to the new situation. In musicians, movement becomes even more important when the goal is trying to break them out of the pattern of the repetitive postures they need to adopt in order to play. While PSE target spinal muscles and posture control, sports activities work the large muscles concerned with limb movements [4].

In order to prevent pain and injury, exercises should be introduced early in life. School screening programs are recommended for the early diagnosis of idiopathic scoliosis. Amongst assessment methodologies Adam's forward bending test associated with a Scoliometer has proved to be a highly useful evaluation tool [6].

Also, the TRACE scale has been recently proposed and validated (a 12 point scale based on a visual assessment of shoulders, scapulae, waist and hemi-thorax asymmetry). Intra-observer repeatability was good, while inter-observer repeatability was poor being the minimum significant change of four [7]. Finally, it is recommended that, during growth, clinical follow-up examinations should be performed at least twice a year [8].

Further research regarding scoliosis is required to support or refute the aforementioned general recommendations [2], especially in the performing arts. However, it is believed that with early detection, the health practitioner, together with the performer, should be able to devise strategies and adapt practice in order to minimise symptoms, to prevent the scoliosis progression and to maximise performance.

References

1. Burwell RG, Dangerfield PH. The NOTOM hypothesis for idiopathic scoliosis: is it nullified by the delayed puberty of female rhythmic gymnasts and ballet dancers with scoliosis? Stud Health Technol Inform. 2002;91:12–4.
2. Negrini S, Aulisa A, Aulisa L, Circo A, Mauroy J, Durmala J, Grivas T, Knott P, Kotwicki T, Maruyama T, Minozzi S, O'Brien J, Papadopoulos D, Rigo M, Rivard C, Romano M, Wynne J, Villagrasa M, Weiss H, Zaina F. 2011 SOSORT guidelines: orthopaedic and rehabilitation treatment of idiopathic scoliosis during growth. Scoliosis. 2012;7:3.
3. Negrini S, Aulisa L, Ferraro C, Fraschini P, Masiero S, Simonazzi P, Tedeschi C, Venturin A. Italian guidelines on rehabilitation treatment of adolescents with scoliosis or other spinal deformities. Eura Medicophys. 2005;41(2):183–201.
4. Stagnara P, Mollon G, De Mauroy J. Reeducation des scolioses. Paris: Expansion Scientifique Francaise; 1990.
5. Meyer C, Cammarata E, Haumont T, Deviterne D, Gauchard G, Leheup B, Lascombes P, Perrin P. Why do idiopathic scoliosis patients participate more in gymnastics? Scand J Med Sci Sports. 2006;16(4):231–6.
6. Bunnell WP. Outcome of spinal screening. Spine. 1993;18(12):1572–80.
7. Zaina F, Negrini S, Atanasio S. TRACE (Trunk Aesthetic Clinical Evaluation), a routine clinical tool to evaluate aesthetics in scoliosis patients: development from the Aesthetic Index (AI) and repeatability. Scoliosis. 2009;4(1):3.
8. Negrini S, Grivas TB, Kotwicki T, Maruyama T, Rigo M, Weiss HR. Why do we treat adolescent idiopathic scoliosis? What we want to obtain and to avoid for our patients. SOSORT 2005 Consensus paper. Scoliosis. 2006;1:4.

Chapter 11
Drugs and Therapeutics

Introduction

This chapter aims to provide a brief overview of the drugs most likely to be encountered in the treatment of performing artists, concentrating on general principles since the drugs available will vary from country to country, according to the licenses that the local regulatory authorities have granted. It is written in simple style so is most likely to appeal to performers, hopefully to educate them in the most rational dosing of any drugs they might need. It may also be of value to health professionals who would not normally be allowed to prescribe drugs or who would not aspire to, but who have the opportunity to educate performers during their relatively long appointments with them. Perhaps even physicians and regular prescribers may also find something of interest.

It should be stressed that in the case of injury, other treatment modalities such as rest and even judicious splinting may be just as effective in pain relief as prescribing a drug and these should always be considered first.

Pharmacokinetics

A drug will only reach the market after comprehensive testing, usually in several countries. By the time it can be purchased there will be extensive documentation available both

H.A. Bird, *Performing Arts Medicine in Clinical Practice*,
DOI 10.1007/978-3-319-12427-8_11,

on its pharmacokinetics (the mathematical modeling of the way it is distributed around the body after absorption) and pharmacodynamics (the way in which it interacts at the cellular level to exert its effect). Some of this is available either as an insert to the package and most can be found on the internet for those prescribers who need this information.

Amongst all of this, the single most useful nugget for the performer is probably a knowledge of the drugs half-life. This is the time it takes for half of the total dose of drug ingested to be excreted from the body. It informs on the frequency of dosing needed and has implications for effective use and for reducing side-effects.

A drug with a half-life of 2–3 h should become active within some 30 min of oral ingestion, will be at its most effective around 2 h after ingestion but may need to be replenished after some 4 h. Such drugs are ideal for giving relief just when it is most needed, perhaps during a rehearsal or during the performance. In turn, if their use is restricted just to that event, the risks of side-effects are correspondingly reduced.

A drug with a half-life of around 6 h may still be effective within the hour but will be at its best around 4 h after ingestion and may have completely worn off after 8 h. So a single dose might cover both rehearsal and performance.

Drugs with half-lives of some 8 h or more are suitable for once daily dosing, if this is more convenient when the symptoms are chronic but the period during which it might exert its side-effects is correspondingly longer so there is much to be said for the use of drugs of short half-life whenever this is possible.

Routes of Administration

Drugs are normally taken by mouth as the easiest and most practical route even though allowance has to be made for the time taken for the drug to pass through the stomach and then the liver. The presence of food in the stomach may slightly delay absorption. For some drugs that are only converted into their active form on passage through the liver, this is the only route available for dosing. The suppository route is a little slower and mainly avoids the liver.

The intra-venous route gives immediate drug action but is clearly not practical. The route of intra-muscular injection has an intermediate speed of action but ensures the drug is delivered to the body, avoiding any vagaries of malabsorption in the stomach which can occasionally occur.

Some analgesics and many anti-inflammatory agents are also available in topical format, that is as a cream or paste that can be rubbed onto the skin. Absorption does occur through the skin but is slower and less reliable than by mouth, though can be enhanced by certain chemicals that are sometimes included into the formulation. The main argument for this route is that the drug "just reaches the spot where it is most needed". The evidence that this is the case is slender and most drugs probably pass around the body soon after absorption through the skin though they may then be preferentially localized at areas of inflammation because they have a good blood supply. That apart, patients divide in their views on this route of delivery. Some benefit form the psychological aspect of being seen to "apply something where it is needed". Others find the preparations cumbersome and messy and a few even have a tendency to stain the clothes.

The intra-lesional or intra-articular injectable routes, for example to a tennis elbow or into a knee or shoulder joint, also both require the use of a syringe and an experienced practitioner with appropriate skills. The drug is theoretically delivered to the site of action, though it is surprising how frequently the required location is missed if the injection is done blind without ultra-sonic or X-ray guidance. How long the drug stays at that site before it travels around the body will depend in part on its size and solubility as well as on the blood supply away from the site.

Analgesics

These relieve pain, from whatever cause, including musculoskeletal pain. They also give some relief from the swelling of inflammation. Table 11.1 shows some common analgesics with their half-lives.

TABLE 11.1 Half life of some common analgesics

Paracetamol	2 h
Pentazocine	2 h
Codeine	3 h
Dihydrocodeine	3 h

The standard choice, time honoured and available over the counter in the UK, is Paracetamol which has a half-life of 2–3 h and which can be taken in divided doses up to 4.0 g a day, normally as two 500 mg tablets every 4 h as required. In this dose there are no major side-effects though very large doses can cause liver failure, even death, which is why there is usually a restriction on the number of tablets that can be purchased at any one time. If paracetamol is needed for more than a few days, and certainly more than a week, medical advice should be sought.

Rarely more potent analgesics are required, such as codeine, but there is never any justification for the strongest opiates such as morphine in performers unless they have other serious disease.

NSAIDs

Non Steroidal Anti-Inflammatory Drugs (NSAIDs) are all distant relatives of aspirin. They relieve inflammation, hence improve fever, as well as reducing the swelling of injury. Partly because of this they relieve pain though they also have a mild analgesic action in their own right. They have been developed from aspirin over last 80 years, initially by the route of the phenylbutazone and then the indomethacin families (Table 11.2).

Nowadays those in routine use are derivatives of ibuprofen, a propionic acid first synthesized in the 1960s, though recently a further group, the coxibs have become available. Although these are a little more specific in relieving inflammation, their association with cardiac side–effects has reduced

Table 11.2 Non-steroidal anti-inflammatory drugs (NSAIDs) classified by family

Aspirin group
Phenylbutazone group
Indomethacin group
Propionic acids
Coxibs

Table 11.3 NSAID side-effects by family

Aspirin: severe gastro-intestinal
Phenylbutazone: marrow depression with potential to cause death
Indomethacin: central nervous system side-effects and fluid retention
Propionic acids: skin rash
Coxibs: cardiovascular events

their use. The specific side effects associated with each of the several groups are shown in Table 11.3.

All NSAID's cause irritation of the stomach and also a very slight reversible reduction in kidney function, both features that the coxibs were designed to prevent. In addition several sometimes cause a mild skin rash.

The oldest drugs of the ibuprofen group have long since lost their patent so generic formulations are available relatively cheaply and moreover in the UK many of these have been licensed for purchase over the counter without prescription from chemists in the high street, though sometimes in doses lower than those that doctors can prescribe.

Within the several NSAIDs that fall into these categories, there is a wide diversity of half-life to cater for all needs (Table 11.4) and the authors preference is to restrict use to this group of 5–6 rather than explore any of the other 30 or so that are available in some countries.

Ibuprofen therefore becomes the usual first choice in a dose of 200 or 400 mg every 4 h up to a very maximum of

TABLE 11.4 Approximate half-lives of some common NSAIDs

Ibuprofen	2 h
Ketoprofen	2 h
Diclofenac	2 h
Aspirin	5 h
Naproxen	12 h
Piroxicam	48 h

2.4 g in any 24 h period. If this causes dyspepsia or other stomach symptoms it may be best to switch to paracetamol rather than to try another. As with that drug, if the ibuprofen is needed for more than 3–4 days a medical opinion should be sought.

Steroid Injections

It is not often realized that there is almost as much diversity between the different steroid preparations available for injection as there is between the many NSAIDs. The performer especially should always enquire exactly what injection is proposed since in performers it is always safest to start with the mildest in the hope that will be sufficiently effective. Dancers, however, may need to start with an initial stronger injection in the leg than an instrumentalist requiring an injection to the hands.

Steroids are the supreme anti-inflammatory drug, and the bodies own means of defense, but they have side effects hence the desirability of developing NSAIDs for longer term routine use. The side effects are many and diverse, especially in those needing to take regular long term oral steroids but for the performer the benefits of the occasional use of a steroid injection, perhaps the only means of allowing continuation at a crucial performance, invariably outweigh the disadvantages. If, however, a performer is resorting to regular

Table 11.5 Intra-articular steroids

Hydrocortisone
Prednisolone and salts
Methylprednisolone
Triamcinolone
Triamcinolone hexacetonide

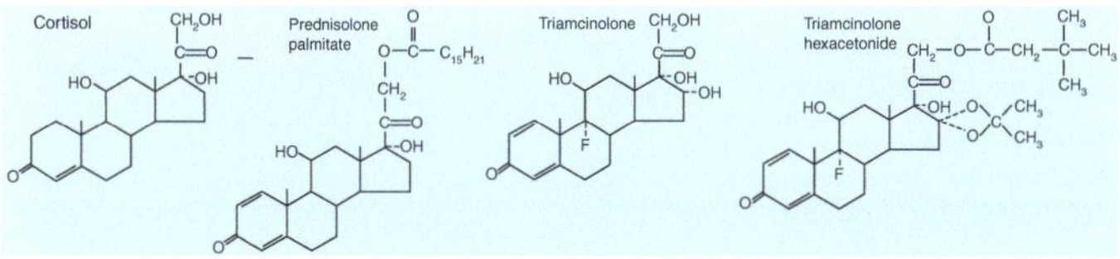

Figure 11.1 Comparative steroid structure (With permission from Elsevier (Hochberg et al. *Rheumatology*. 3rd ed. Mosby; 2003))

steroid injections, a firm diagnosis and alternative treatment options should always be sought.

Many anti-inflammatory steroids exist (Table 11.5) of varying chemical structure (Fig. 11.1). The "natural" steroid is hydrocortisone, the mildest and least harmful of the group and probably the injection of choice for the fragile extensor tendon sheaths in the hands of musicians. Prednisolone is a stronger synthetic analogue but has rather more side-effects. It can be formulated as one of several salts which reduce the solubility conferring greater local potency (Table 11.6). The prednisolone molecule can also be manipulated to give methylprednisolone or triamcinolone, by the addition of a fluorine atom, progressively giving greater activity but an even greater risk of side-effects. When six side chains are added to the hyperactive triamcinolone to make it much less soluble as triamcinolone hexacetonide, the result is a steroid that has such a potent capacity for local tissue damage that it has been banned in most countries. Since there is a range of permissible doses for each of these steroids the precise choice

TABLE 11.6 Comparative steroid solubility and duration of action (With permission from Elsevier (Hochberg et al. Rheumatology. 3rd ed. Mosby; 2003))

Preparation	Relative doses required to provide equivalent pharmacological effect	Average duration of pain relief (days)	Solubility[a]
Hydrocortisone acetate	×6.5	6.0	0.0018
Hydrocortisone *tert*-butyl acetate	×6.25	12.1	–
Prednisolone acetate	×5	7.8	–
Prednisolone *tert*-butyl acetate	×5	14.5	<0.0010
6-methylprednisolone acetate	×5	8.2	0.0014
Dexamethasone acetate	1	7.6	–
Dexamethasone *tert*-butyl acetate	1	14.9	–
Triamcinolone diacetonide	×5	7.7	0.0056
Triamcinolone acetonide	×5	14.2	0.0040
Triamcinolone hexacetonide	×5	21.2	0.0004

[a]Percentage w/v in H_2O at 25 °C

of optimum drug and dose for each individual pathology and performer becomes an art form in itself!

One useful ploy is to use one of the mildest short-acting steroids to confirm an inflammatory diagnosis when it becomes more justifiable to follow this up with a second more potent and longer acting steroid to provide the cure.

Stage Fright

This affects many performers at some stage during their career. Dancers seem to find it less of a problem that instrumentalists, singers or actors. This may be partly because dancers are usually active when on stage and can exercise when off it. The orchestral musician, although an athlete of the arms, has to sit still until required. Under-rehearsal or lack of confidence with the technicalities of a particularly difficult part often contribute. Social factors like nicotine or even recreational drugs may aggravate and alcohol as a remedy is not always beneficial.

This author believes that a psychological approach to the problem is invariably the best and that the use of drugs, such as the "beta-blockers" should be avoided in view of their side effects. Figures on the proportion of performers who resort to these at some stage of their career are hard to verify and it is salutary to consider that most obtain them form friends of order them from the internet when problems of product purity may also be an issue. One survey has suggested that some 27 % of American orchestral players may have used them at some stage.

This author believes that the main thrust of treatment should be through expert psychological advice and counselling, rather than with the use of drugs.

Beta-adrenoceptor blocking drugs or "beta-blockers" have a specific effect on the sympathetic nervous system. Thus they have no effect on emotional factors that might aggravate stage fright but improve the physiological features of anxiety such as rapid heart rate, sweating, fast breathing and tremor. If tremor is impeding performance, that performance is likely to be improved but the drive may be lost. Thus they also improve performance in archery and shooting so are banned drugs for these sports.

Minor side-effects with all of the drugs include dizziness, tiredness, diarrhoea and blurred vision, but the major issue is the tendency of certain of them to act on the lungs to cause spasm of the airways and therefore to cause or aggravate asthma in susceptible individuals. Those that cause this can cause serious illness, even death from respiratory arrest, which is why the drugs should only be prescribed by a doctor after a full risk assessment. They are also contra-indicated in some subjects with slow heart rates and those that enter the nervous system also have a tendency to cause nightmares.

Because of this a few advocate the use of anxiolytic drugs such as diazepam as an alternative, which are sometimes prescribed for anxiety state and even sleeplessness. However, they tend to be addictive and can relax muscles which is clearly disadvantageous to performers.

Medication for Singers

Singers, along with brass and wind players, require attention to the vocal apparatus as well in addition to musculo-skeletal care. A trained singer or actor, however, employs tricks to use an impaired vocal apparatus in a more efficient manner, so simple respiratory ailments often do not to have as much impact on the voice as would occur without such training.

The discipline of singing can assist chronic conditions such as asthma and in the management of the acute infection there may be a role for mucolytics and cough suppressants in moderation though expectorants are felt to mainly exert a placebo effect.

An under-appreciated problem in elite singers is that of reflux gastric dyspepsia connected with the use of their intra-abdominal pressure and diaphragm both of which serve to project gastric acidity upwards if the gastric sphincter is lax or inefficient. This may require treatment by conventional means.

Chapter 12
The Disabled Performer

Introduction

At first sight, physical disability, especially one involving the musculo-skeletal system, would seem to be a disadvantage for the performer, particularly for one in the professional category. This may also be more true of dancers than of musicians. This chapter refutes that supposition, by reference to the case histories of two musicians. The first describes the expertise needed for the rehabilitation of a professional trumpeter who had an acute stroke. The second describes a folk singer and guitarist who proceeded to a near full time career after an accident that transected his spinal cord. Finally a dance company is discussed that innovatively employs disabled dancers alongside those without disability.

A Trumpeter with a Stroke

EM, born in 1962, played the trumpet, cornet and trombone but the trumpet was his main instrument with which he led his own concert salsa band. He also played as a locum in orchestras as well as performing some solo work and giving lessons.

In May 2010, 5 min into giving his first trumpet lesson of the day and allegedly as a result of hitting his first high note

H.A. Bird, *Performing Arts Medicine in Clinical Practice*,
DOI 10.1007/978-3-319-12427-8_12,

of the day, he collapsed with a stroke, affecting his left cerebral cortex. He was immediately transferred to a specialist hospital where investigations suggested this was haemorrhagic rather than occlusive. He received excellent and comprehensive care under the National Health Service in the UK, and was judged by their rehabilitation team to have made an excellent recovery.

Understandably and interestingly, this expert team did not have all the skills required to allow him to return to his previous career. He considered he was left with three persistent problems, all relatively minor but each critical to his playing and therefore sought an opinion from a Performing Arts Medicine clinic on whether anything further could be done.

First, the slight residual weakness in the right arm, although not compromising activities of daily living, specifically "weakened" the ring finger on the valve of the trumpet, the middle and index fingers on the adjacent valves both unaffected. Careful examination of the ring finger actually showed power and tone to be normal and the inter-phalangeal joins functioned normally. There was however, a clear deficit in proprioception in the lower half of finger excursion when the valve was depressed, that impeded his performance. So specific and localised, this was presumed to be cortical in origin. The hand physiotherapists concerned were advised to concentrate on re-training proprioception rather than power, in so far that this was possible.

Second, weakness of the facial musculature and therefore the embouchure, which restricted playing to 30 min at a stretch, was aggravated by a specific loss of sensation in the anterior third of the tongue, perhaps also with some minor motor deficit in the tongue. This further restricted his ability to tongue rapidly repeated "flutter" notes. He was advised that this sensation might not return and in collaboration with colleagues, he devised a new method to tongue "flutter" notes using other parts of the tongue.

Third, and most intriguing, he was experiencing problems with cortical perception, only revealed in relation to the demanding requirements of professional music making at this level. Sight reading had suddenly become more difficult. Although he had not lost his sense of pitch, he was now unable to distinguish a minor key from the major key at the same pitch by ear. He was also unable to cue the exact entries of the other band members, especially when they were standing to his left. This was because he could no longer anticipate their entry points, rather than because of any muscular deficit. This required the delegation of this task to others.

With adjustments to technique and with some delegation, he was however able to return to the majority of his previous activities in terms of playing.

A Guitarist with Spinal Cord Transection

TD, born in 1957, was involved in a motor cycle road traffic accident in 1974, which caused a major fracture of the sixth cervical vertebra but also a lesser fracture at the seventh and at several of the upper thoracic vertebrae as well. As a result the spinal cord was transected, probably partially at several levels around this area, such that he was confined to a wheelchair but had substantial use of both arms and hands.

Interestingly, and in spite of this disability he subsequently decided to give up his job as a mental health administrator and to become a professional musician. Previously an amateur, he had been a folk singer accompanying himself on the guitar. It was impossible for him to stand and the wheelchair did not allow use of a conventional guitar so he switched to a steel lap guitar. He had performed professionally for some 10 years (Figs. 12.1 and 12.2).

His performances involved a combination of singing and playing, usually together. His income was mainly derived from this act but he did some composing so also received licensing fees. He was able to play easily for some 15 min but might then become restricted by cramp, whereupon he would switch to singing while an assistant, who often travelled with him, would come on stage and massage his shoulders. He had a website and a fan club.

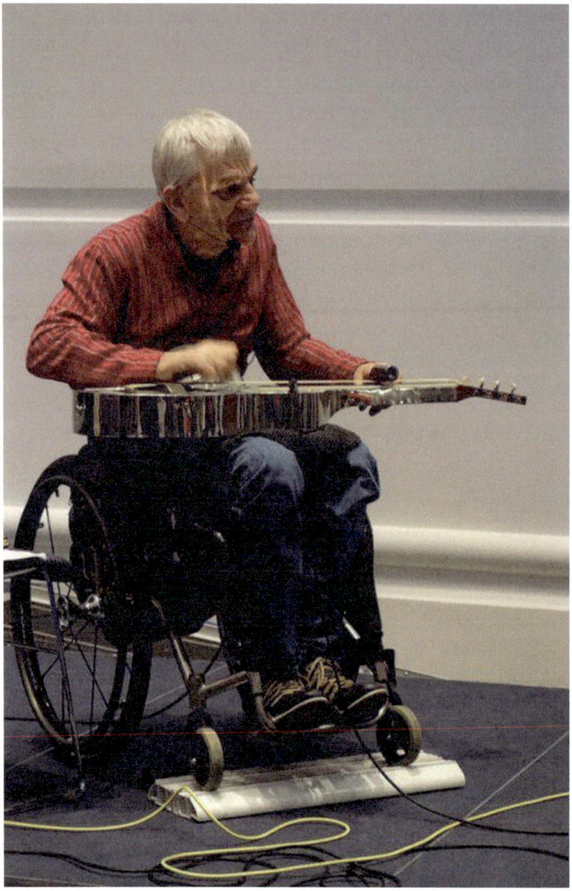

FIGURE 12.1 TD with lap guitar

In his stage career, spanning many years, there had been several medical issues resulting from the site of the injury, which were complex and beyond the scope of this chapter. Serial MRI scans had confirmed that there was a syrinx in the spinal cord at the level of C6 and there was also some secondary atrophy of the cord above and below this. Some of his symptoms therefore resembled syringomyelia. At one point

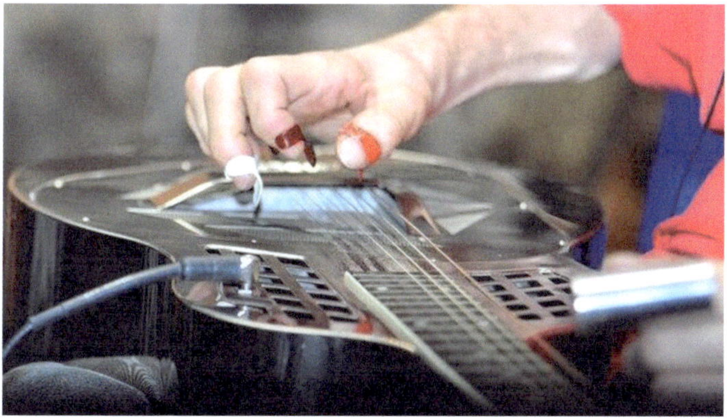

FIGURE 12.2 Adaptions made to the fingers

an infected spinal facet joint had been suspected but since there was convincing secondary degenerative change at most of the vertebrae that had fractured, it seems likely that this may have been a local area of inflammation, secondary to the degeneration.

Perhaps also as a result of the accident there was an antero-listhetic slip of C4 on C5 and a consequent narrowing of the right C4/C5 foramen, aggravated by a disc bulge, which intermittently compressed the right C5 nerve root at its exit foramen. This might have been one of the main causes of the right shoulder and sometimes arm pain that he experienced, though others had judged it neuropathic in that it responded to pregabalin. However other features of that pain suggested mechanical overuse, the pain sometimes relieved by stretching, and also position dependent, though in part this probably reflected the contorted position of the neck he increasingly needed to adopt to continue playing his lap guitar (Fig. 12.3).

In spite of all these adversities, he has courageously continued to tackle and overcome them all in pursuit of his chosen career with a combination of pressure point relief, acupuncture, therapeutic ultrasound and manipulation.

Further information available at: www.tomdoughty.com.

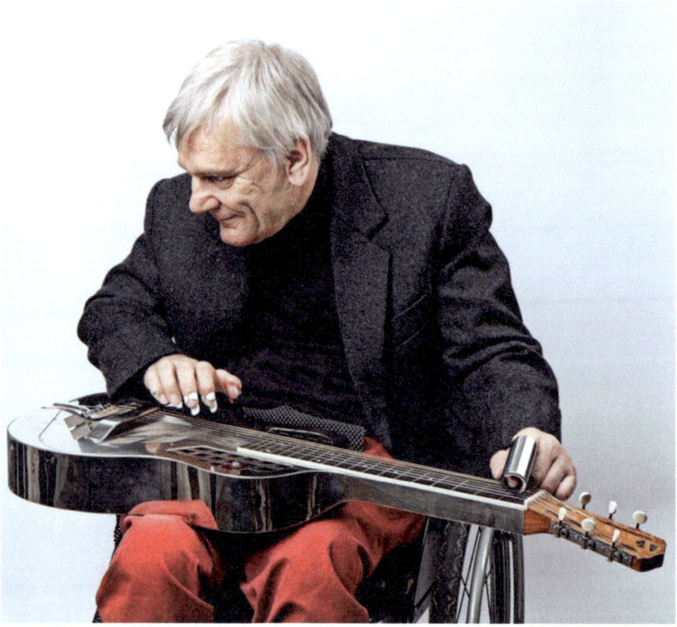

FIGURE 12.3 The position required of the neck

Candoco

Candoco (Can do company) is the name of an enterprising UK Contemporary Dance Company that was founded in 1991 by Celeste Dandeker and Adam Benjamin after the former had sustained an injury on stage while performing that rendered her paraplegic. Initially anticipating a complete retirement from dance, she was persuaded to return to the stage by Darshan Singh Buller, the choreographer, dancing from a wheel chair. This was the inspiration for the founding of the company.

The company performs a wide range of contemporary dance using both disabled dancers and non-disabled dancers (Fig. 12.4).

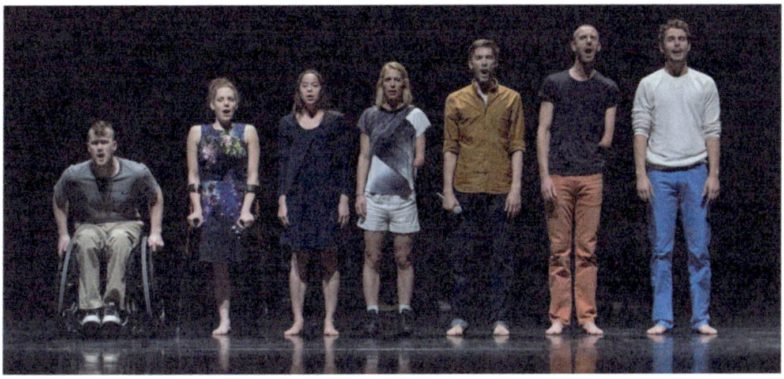

FIGURE 12.4 Candoco Dance Company 2014/15 (Photographer Hugo Glendinning. www.candoco.co.uk)

They use world class choroegraphers to devise a wide repertoire and have extensive learning and development projects and opportunities.

Their web site states their philosophy: "We are a passionate dedicated team of people and we want to show you what dance can be and who can dance."

Further information available at: www.candoco.co.uk.

Chapter 13
The Multi-Talented Performer

Introduction

Many performers are expert in more than one genre. For the free-lance dancer it is likely to be advantageous at audition to perform in many different dance styles. Instrumentalists may also be versatile in more than one instrument. Musical Conservatoires invariably require a "second instrument" to be specified when auditioning for a "first instrument". This facility may also be of use in a saturated job market or for teaching purposes. Some conservatoires offer mixed courses combining dance with music with theatre. In addition many performing artists, especially dancers, maintain an interest in sport, particularly tariff sports such as gymnastics, cheerleading and diving.

For performers who also have musculo-skeletal problems, this can create difficulties in management especially where participation in one activity aggravates the injuries caused by another or delays their healing. The medical priorities of the clinician are not always those of the performer!

An applied area of particular importance is the multi-talented adolescent, perhaps already with injury problems who could proceed with equal ease either to an instrument or to dance. The clinician is sometimes called upon to give an opinion on which genre is likely to be injury free.

H.A. Bird, *Performing Arts Medicine in Clinical Practice*,
DOI 10.1007/978-3-319-12427-8_13,

This chapter discusses three illustrative case histories that fall within this area, one of which has appeared briefly before in the chapter on scoliosis but which appears here in more detail.

A Dancer Who Played the Cello

As a child KB, born in 1981, was equally talented at dance and music. She described herself as self-driven at both with a desire to excel. Musically she loved and played the cello with piano as her subsidiary instrument. In dance she excelled at ballet, helped to a large extent by her inherited joint hyperlaxity. She continued seriously both with ballet, adding modern dance, until the age of 13 and with her cello until the age of 15. There was considerable speculation within the family as to which of these genres might form the basis of her future career.

She danced to such a high standard that application to a national ballet school was considered. With her cello she performed in the regional youth orchestra attached to the regional music conservatoire. In view of her musical talent, she was bequeathed a valuable antique cello by an admirer.

Since childhood she had suffered both from migraine, perhaps indicative of her desire to excel and from musculoskeletal symptoms, particularly back pain that were largely relieved by her dancing. However, and probably reasonably, lay opinion was that with her joint symptoms, a career as a cellist might be the safer option with less propensity to injury than a career as a dancer. She was encouraged to concentrate exclusively on her cello and gave up her dance. Unfortunately, at this time she developed a painful ganglion at the right wrist, perhaps reflecting her hyperlaxity. The local general practitioner in the rural area where she lived referred to a local well-intentioned orthopaedic surgeon who enthusiastically removed the ganglion and later repaired a torn ligament at the same wrist.

As a result of these two operations she was left with an extremely stiff right wrist (her bowing arm), which severely restricted her ability to bow and essentially brought her serious playing career to an end. In spite of multiple attempts to return to the instrument, she had to give up all her aspirations to a career as a soloist and enrolled at university for a theoretical musical degree with the piano as her instrument of choice.

She completed her degree and for a time taught music and the piano, whilst also working as a nursing auxiliary to supplement her income. She still aspired to the cello and when she became aware of a recently established Performing Arts Medicine clinic she self appointed and sought career advice.

By now back pain was the main problem and the investigations that revealed both a mild scoliosis and Schmorl's nodes are described in Chap. 9 where there are also illustrations of her X-rays. As a result of intensive physiotherapy and activity including a return to dance, combined with appropriate analgesia, the nodes healed and she left her job as a nursing auxiliary for a more secure post in university administration. From this post she played a large part in initiating and facilitating the inauguration of the British Association for Performing Arts Medicine's student advocate scheme. Here she piloted a counseling service for music students with medical difficulties arising from their playing.

After a gap of some 15 years she has recently returned to cello playing with a Yamaha SVC 210 electronic cello (Fig. 13.1), preferred to the classical cello for several reasons. It is lighter and can be easily twisted while playing as she compensates for the disadvantage of the slight twist in her spine. She has been advised that if foot pedals are used to amplify the sound these should never be fixed in relation to the cello, which would tend to fix the pelvis and negate this advantage. She has also discovered that the income procured from playing this instrument in a popular repertoire far exceeds the income procured from the classical cello.

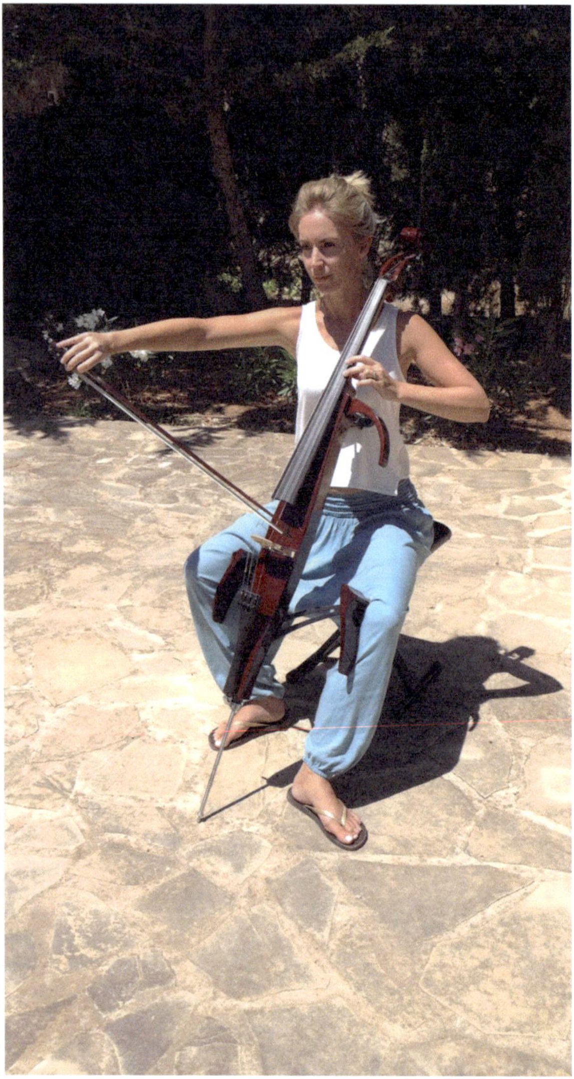

FIGURE 13.1 Electronic cello played by KB

Piano or Ballet?

AF, born in 1988, was a music student at University with the piano as her main instrument but was also secretary of the University Dance Society. That reflected her two main loves throughout childhood; ballet and the piano. Medical problems had hitherto been minor. At the age of 18 she had some pain and swelling, just in the right hand, later in the arm and neck, after playing for some 15 min. Living in London, this patient had easy access to a specialist Performing Arts clinic, where she was seen by an expert. Spasm was noted in both trapeziae, presumed from overuse, and physiotherapy was recommended which resolved the problem though she had to cancel her piano performers diploma examination.

She soldiered on for some 4 years reaching the author at a Performing Arts Clinic close to her University in June 2010. Now in her final year at university, she still aspired to retake her diploma at the same time she took her degree using much the same repertoire for the diploma as for her final degree recital.

The earlier symptoms remained in abeyance, but a different type of pain in both hands and forearms had occurred, specifically only caused by the final movement of the Ravel Sonatine. As a result she had hardly played at all for the previous 2 months.

On examination there was a clear tendonitis affecting the extensor tendons of the middle, ring and little finger on the right hand with less marked clinical features at the same tendons in the left hand. So for a second time, with a second trained observer, unilateral features were apparent in an instrument that is predominantly symmetric. Her fingers were hyperlax and there was slight unequal winging of the scapulae. The spine was extremely hypermobile, partly reflecting her dancing prowess, but probably also inherited in view of the laxity at her finger joints which would not have been achieved through dance training.

Investigations were ordered which showed normal haematology and biochemistry, normal acute phase reactants and normal serology, all suggesting any synovitis arose from local mechanical factors rather than from more widespread autoimmune disease.

X-rays (Figs. 13.2, 13.3 and 13.4) were reported as normal apart from a slight listhetic slip at C5. More detailed scrutiny showed that this produced an overall slight lordosis between C6 and C7 and raised the possibility of a mild "S" shaped scoliosis within the thoracic spine, concave to the right between T8 and T12. This might account for the tendency of the symmetric instrument to produce asymmetric symptoms.

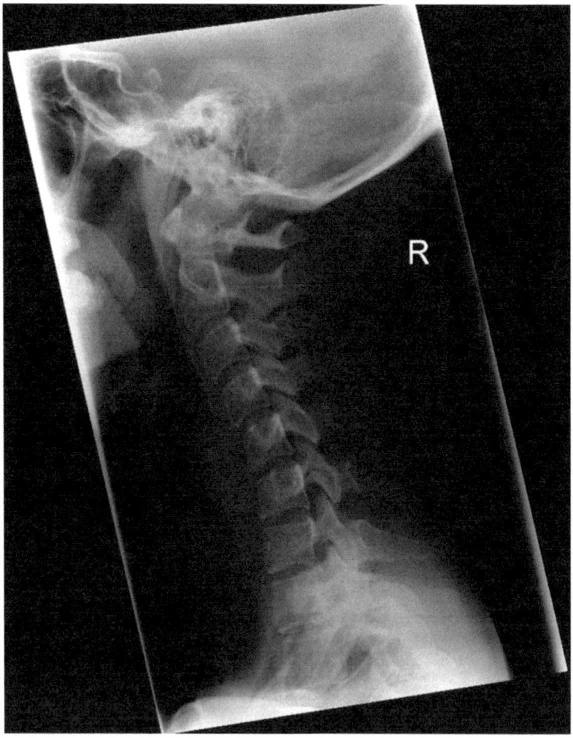

FIGURE 13.2 Lateral X-ray of cervical spine

At follow up and in the light of these, she played part of her repertoire and was advised on how to make a cautious return to the piano. The repertoire was reviewed and it was agreed how those parts of the pieces that were felt likely to aggravate any synovitis would be introduced more gradually. A letter was prepared for the university explaining the medical position and asking for tolerance in the marking of the recital sections that were still causing her difficulty on medical grounds. The diploma should be delayed until after the university exam.

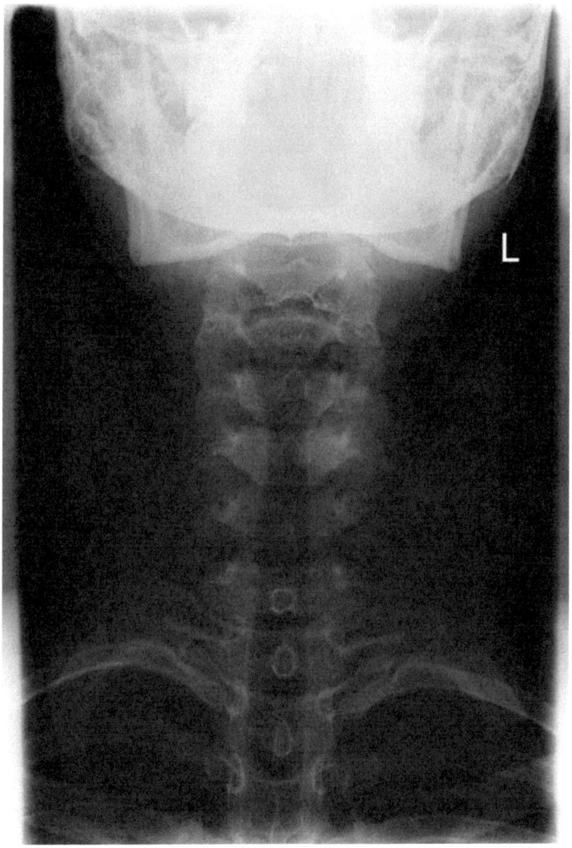

FIGURE 13.3 PA X-ray of cervical spine

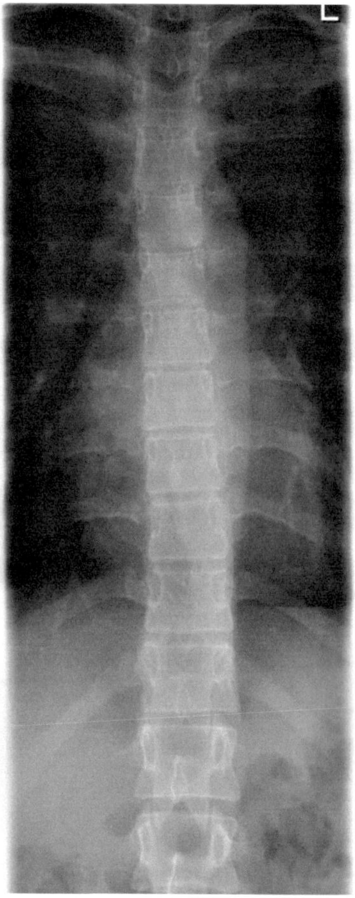

FIGURE 13.4 PA X-ray of thoracic spine

So far, so good. At this point near the end of the consultation she announced that she actually proposed a career in dance! Her parents did not know this and might be annoyed. Neither did her teachers in the music department nor her piano teacher. She had already decided not to inform the music department of her career intentions, but was simultaneously having regular dancing lessons and was already entered for advanced ballet exams.

The needs for these were next considered. It seemed that although she needed forearm strengthening for dance, especially for contemporary, this could also be beneficial in moderation for her piano playing, but if excessive might aggravate her symptoms.

After some discussion it was agreed that the piano recital should still have top priority so that she had a degree under her belt. The piano diploma could wait and the ballet exams should be postponed.

When seen at follow-up 1 year later, she had completed her music degree, postponed her piano diploma examination and completed most of her dance examinations. Her new complaint was of pain at the back of her hyperlax right knee since her return to dance.

At attempted e-mail follow up 1 year later still, she was not available but was thought to be in South America where her parents were now domiciled.

The Violin and Sport

UN, born in 1988, was also multi-talented as a child. Initially taught ballet and tap dancing from the age of 3, she was also sporty, enjoying swimming and kayaking. Music, however, was her main interest and from the age of 14 this was given priority. Violin was her main instrument and she obtained her performers diploma at the age of 17, but alongside this she obtained grade 8 of the Associated Board examinations when she was in the sixth form. In 2007 she started a BMus performers course in violin at University and having attended one of the author's lectures on musicians ailments, she sought his advice at a Performing Arts clinic.

With violin her main instrument and kayaking, performed at a national level, now her main hobby she was experiencing pain in the neck and back, both aggravated by exercise. This was impeding her violin playing. Further, an injury to the shoulder caused by kayaking had rendered her shoulder less stable which was impeding her violin playing.

With unexplained stretch marks and spontaneous skin bruising from the age of 7, bilateral calcaneal apophysitis at the age of 9 and bilateral Osgood Schlatters disease at the age of 11, it was later appreciated that she was hypermobile, her spine especially supple with a tendency to hinge in the mid-lumbar region.

On examination, she was hypermobile in her fingers, thumbs and lumbar spine where she hinged at L2. The left shoulder had a tendency to dislocate but she was able to control this with better than average muscular power, perhaps endowed by her kayaking prowess.

On investigation, haematology, acute phase reactants and serology were all normal. X-rays of the shoulders were entirely normal and other X-rays (Figs. 13.5, 13.6, 13.7 and 13.8) were also reported as normal but the postural forward curve of the cervical spine was unusual and there was a suspicion of a slight “S” shaped twist within the thoracic spine, the mid-point of which accorded with the site of most of her back symptoms.

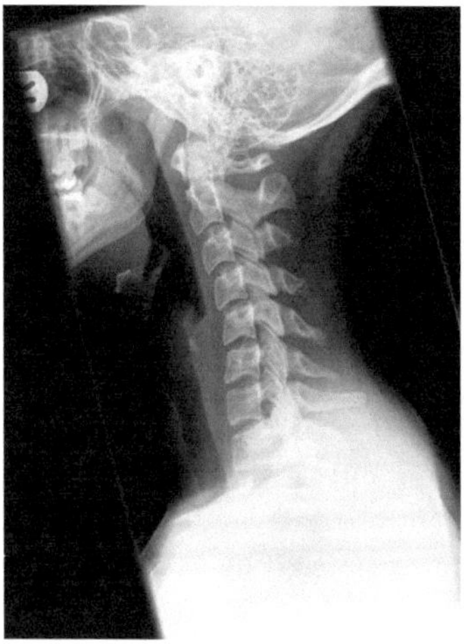

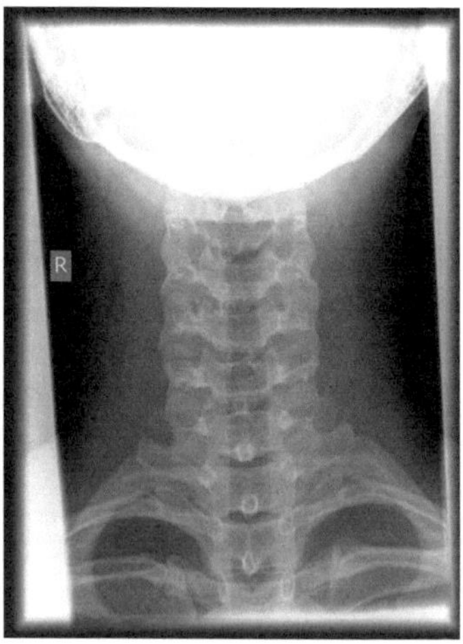

Figures 13.5 and 13.6 X-ray of cervical spine

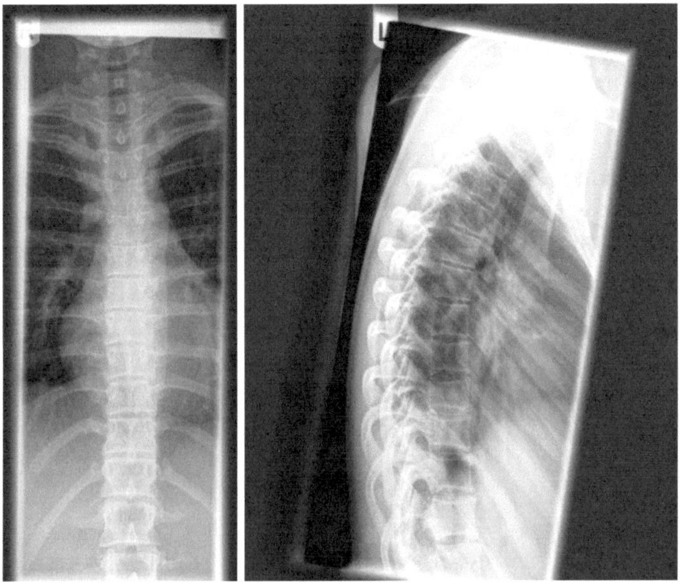

FIGURES 13.7 AND 13.8 X-ray of thoracic spine

Her wish list was that her pain should be relieved and her hyperlaxity better controlled, whilst continuing with both her violin playing and her kayaking. She was reluctant to switch from violin to piano or from kayaking to swimming but both could be an option.

Conventional advice might have been to introduce the Alexander Technique and advise against kayaking until her music degree was completed. However she found the Alexander Technique a little tame and insisted on kayaking. This she modified, however, by a switch from the demanding white water kayaking (analogous to a contact sport) to kayak polo where there is a need for similar strength but in which the environment is more predictable so the risk of injury such as sudden dislocation, much less.

After much consideration she did transfer from the performers course to a more theoretical musicology course although this caused her considerable emotional trauma at the time. Here she also achieved, awarded the best first class honours degree for some years, in large part for her research dissertation on Joint Hypermobility in Musicians.

Currently she is completing a PhD and also acts as the national co-ordinator for the British Association of Performing Arts Medicine student advocate scheme that was inaugurated a decade earlier by the first subject of this chapter.

Discussion

The first case illustrates the difficulties of career selection in a multi-talented performer with minor musculo-skeletal problems who lives in an area where there is no immediate access to Performing Arts Medicine. The suggestion of her parents to their offspring that the cello would be a "safer" choice than dance is quite understandable. The benign nature of the ganglion, common in joint hypermobility where it is usually induced by mechanical stress so is possibly protective was not fully appreciated by the general practitioner. The enthusiastic surgery, always a risk in the hands and arms of musicians might have been more restrained and it is probable the surgeon did not fully appreciate the need for flexibility in the bowing wrist of a cellist, where extreme stability is not required.

We can only speculate on whether, had career advice been sought from an expert at the age of 13, she would have been advised to concentrate on a career in dance rather than with the cello, on the basis that the hyperlax shoulders would have been an advantage and the spinal curve would not have disadvantaged with the discipline of the regular exercise. Such advice for the multi-talented adolescent is an important but relatively neglected area of Performing Arts Medicine although in tis case would have required a practitioner with knowledge of both instrumental and dance medicine.

Both the first two cases illustrate the ease with which some artists can move from one genre to another. But if the first illustrates determination, the second perhaps illustrates more the "artistic temperament" with its capacity to change tack precipitously, coupled with the tendency of some artists to set themselves almost unrealistic targets. Perhaps, if it becomes apparent that these targets may not be achieved, this can lead to disappointment verging on frustration, aggravating the tendency to want to change course.

The second case also raises some moral dilemmas. Ultimately a doctors obligation is to their patient, all aspects of the consultation remaining confidential. However there has to be a certain sympathy for the university, always supportive of their student though perhaps not kept fully in the picture.

The third case emphasizes the links between sports medicine and science and the performing arts. Although dancers perhaps have a greater tendency to involve themselves in all sports related to movement, musicians also play sports in their recreational time. At first sight the combination of elite violin playing with white water kayaking in a subject who has hyperlax subluxing shoulders seems to provide a particular challenge. However the subject had great insight into both activities and was able to adapt each such that they became complementary in their effect, the shoulder strengthening provided by the sport protecting and stabilizing the bowing arm. Ultimately, however, she made the transition from the most extreme style of kayaking and from the most demanding type of violin playing to find academic achievement and satisfaction in other areas. As one door closes another door opens.

Chapter 14
Future Trends

Introduction

The preface and Chap. 1 briefly allude to recent initiatives in developing the speciality of Performing Arts Medicine. In the UK, these include the longstanding clinical work of BAPAM (British Association for Performing Arts Medicine) and the more recent Healthier Dancer programme of Dance UK as well as the MSc degree in Performing Arts Medicine at University College, London, now in its fourth year at the time of writing.

This chapter briefly reviews progress already made and then attempts to peer into the future, speculating on what is still needed and what might be most feasible. It will also review important new initiatives such as the Musical Impact project, currently funded by the Arts and Humanities Research Council in the UK.

Ultimately it is a personal viewpoint although one that has been influenced by years of experience, albeit mainly in the UK.

BAPAM

The British Association for Performing Arts Medicine commenced life as the Elmdon Trust, founded by the late Dr Ian James, a clinical pharmacologist at the Royal Free Hospital in

H.A. Bird, *Performing Arts Medicine in Clinical Practice*,
DOI 10.1007/978-3-319-12427-8_14,

London who was also an accomplished viola player and who researched the death of Mozart. He started a musicians clinic in 1984 and suffering from stage fright himself, he inaugurated the first controlled trials of beta adrenergic drugs for musicians. In 1989 the organization became the British Performing Arts Medicine Trust and subsequently became BAPAM.

Early luminaries were the late Christopher Wynn-Parry (a rehabilitationist) and Ian Winspur (a hand surgeon). Subsequently the late Justin Howse, Rodney Grahame, and Mike Shipley amongst others, have all played important roles. Traditionally the organisation has attracted doctors who are also amateur musicians though later other practitioners, especially physiotherapists, have become involved.

The practitioners directory thus still lists a majority of doctors alongside examples of most other specialist practitioners that have ever been of value to the speciality. Regular clinics are held in consulting rooms at their central London offices and there is also a network of regular but less frequent provincial clinics. Any performer can phone and request an appointment, the first diagnostic assessment free, since most practitioners do not charge for their time. Any subsequent treatment recommended is often provided through the organization at reduced private practice rates. Some practitioners request that the General Practitioners of the most complex cases refer the performer to their NHS practices from which further investigations can be arranged. The organization is regulated to perfection and all practitioners are required to submit an application for consideration and then to attend regular training which is provided by BAPAM either free or at a reduced commercial rate.

At present well over 80 % of all performers attending are musicians. Dancers and actors account for most of the rest though even circus is represented. Appointments are booked centrally, wherever possible with someone with at least some expertise in that particular genre. In spite of this satisfaction is high on attendee feedback and most performers appreciate the normal 30 min appointment time with someone who shows sympathy. Professionally, the lack of easy access to diagnostic facilities and the lack of access to subsequent follow-up care can be slightly frustrating.

Other activities are educational including the provision of patient information material and acting as a partner with University College London in the establishment of the MSc in Performing Arts Medicine. Students enrolled on this course attend BAPAM teaching clinics. A student advocate scheme has also been piloted in the school of music at the University of Leeds and is now being rolled out nationally. It also publishes a house journal electronically.

Dance UK

Almost simultaneously, Dance UK was founded in 1981. It has a wider brief than BAPAM and acts partly as an agency to facilitate the career of dancers who pay an annual membership fee for the services it provides. It is proud of its strong political voice and to some extent, acts as a trade union for dancers from all genres. It works hard to encourage greater sponsorship of all aspects of dance. Educational workshops and career advice are both provided. A register of expert speakers is maintained, who are available to teach in various dance institutions.

Arguably a jewel in the crown, the Healthier Dancer Programme, was developed significantly from around 2008, and is the part of the organization most relevant to this book. It provides education material for dancers of all genres and supports and encourages research in the speciality. A practitioners register is maintained, covering all aspects of health care that can be consulted on the organisation's web-site without the need for membership of Dance UK. Perhaps reflecting the aims and origins of the organization, only a very small proportion of the practitioners are doctors; many are physiotherapists, osteopaths, chiropracters, nutritionists and psychologists though all therapy types even those distantly represented to dance, are represented. Appointments are not arranged; the performer contacts the practitioner directly and only dancers are seen though "dance" is interpreted in the widest sense so cheerleaders and circus would also be welcome. Formal practitioner training is not at present provided (though is being considered) and placement on the register is through recommendation by previous patients. A small number of practitioners, including the author, are on both registers.

Recently a new National Institute for Dance Medicine and Science (NIDMS) has been established at the Royal National Orthopaedic Hospital's central London site, the hospital combining with six major dance institutions or universities to provide easy and rapid access dance clinics which are of particular value to freelance dancers or those dancing with most of the small companies that can not afford their own medical support. Investigational facilities are available through the hospital, the system ultimately largely funded from the NHS from general Practitioner budgets though donations from industry and individuals are encouraged. It is anticipated that this will act as a springboard for research into dance medicine.

NHS Clinics

These contrasting approaches to the care of performers, both models having evolved over some years, illustrate some of the difficulties in the provision of care for performers. Both apply in the context of a country that has a nationalised health service, that has recently adopted a greater element of an "internal market", in which private health care is also easily available, but where it is still not the norm.

In countries where health care is provided mainly or exclusively in the private sector, funded by insurance, expensive easy and immediate access to medical care for as long an appointment as is needed does not represent a problem. The main issue is that the average performer is unlikely to be in receipt of a salary that will allow this and a minor issue is that the practitioner is not guaranteed to have expertise in the field.

In countries like the UK where medical care is still largely funded by the state through taxation, access to expert care is theoretically free but unlikely to be immediate. Increasingly, with the development of an internal market, performers risk being elbowed out in preference for what many would feel were important claims such as the treatment of cancer. Time with the primary care physician, once obtained is likely to be limited, perhaps to 5–10 min, even if they possess the expertise to remedy the problem. Alternate attendance at a hospital casualty under the guise of an injury is likely to be even more frustrating.

It remains to be seen whether a model like NIDMS will become sufficiently self supporting for continued success. Meanwhile the system of self-referral, though a charitable organization like BAPAM has much to commend it.

The Leeds Template

Some aspects of the author's provincial experience in Leeds have already been outlined in previous chapters. His appointment with the university, was only part NHS funded allowing access for time to teach and research. This, in turn, allowed a greater freedom than with an NHS appointment alone. When the first local Performing Arts clinics were introduced it was less contentious to do this within the university framework as a teaching, even research exercise. This even allowed the author to organize and book his own clinics, expediting assessment and treatment for performers without friction in the NHS.

The inaugural dance clinics were established within the partner organization the Northern School of Contemporary Dance using their own physiotherapy treatment suite, with the support of the Principal, Nadine Senior. Informal contact with her deputy, Alison Beckett, who was then director of research spawned research projects with a medial slant, leading to co-supervision and often publication.

The inaugural music clinics were established within the school of music at the University, adapting the seminar room and leading to the allocation of a room for Alexander Technique.

For complex patients at either site, transfer to his hospital NHS clinic was requested, with an appropriate letter of request from the (usually) local GP, who was often known personally by the author.

At the school of music the process was facilitated, even reinforced by the inauguration of the student advocate scheme, already described. It soon became apparent, however, that there was a paucity of clinicians adequately trained to deal with the complexities of performers.

The MSc Degree at University College, London

This degree course, long an ambition of BAPAM, took its first students in September 2011 and has since run for 4 years at the time of writing. A search committee from BAPAM considered the large number of possible venues before entering negotiations with the University concerned. For the first such course in the UK, possibly in Europe, the chances of success seemed best in the capital. University College, London, had its own medical school and offered a galaxy of lecturing talent in spite of some concern that their fees might be too much for practitioners in the speciality. For taught masters degrees, Universities set their own fees independently so there can be considerable variation in cost between different Universities. Even if this has been the case, there has still been a constant stream of applicants even though the UCL entry requirements are quite stringent.

Interestingly only some 10 % of these have come from doctors. Most have come from physiotherapists, osteopaths and chiropracters. The course offers instrumental medicine, dance medicine and vocal medicine. It was not clear which would prove most attractive and most applicants have been keen to learn about all three areas. However, the majority already have expertise in dance medicine and have been keen to take this further though for some the research component which accounts for some 30 % of the marks and which has the potential to groom for an MPhil or even a PhD has proved a big attraction. Consideration is currently being given to the creation of a cheaper diploma, just taught in one of the three areas, perhaps with easier entry requirements, that might even attract some performers.

At an early stage the need for partner organisations, selected from amongst the conservatoires, was appreciated. For music, the Royal College of Music where Professor Aaron Williamon had already established the first course in Music Science in the country, was an obvious choice. For dance, Trinity-Laban where Dr Emma Redding had for many years been running the first of the many Dance Science courses in the capital, was an equally obvious choice. This has led both to an interchange with technique teachers and the development of collaborative research.

Research Outlets

A fundamental requirement for research is that it should be disseminated, traditionally either by presentation at meetings of learned societies of by publication either in print or electronically.

For presentation and networking, several international societies exist, each of which holds regular meetings, typically once a year. For dance medicine IADMS (International Association for Dance Medicine and Science), initially with European, even UK ancestry, is pre-eminent. For instrumental medicine the American PAMA (Performing Arts Medicine Association) might be preferred. Both these societies produce their own journals. Others such as ISSTIP (International Society for the Study of Tension in Performance), which also produces a journal but which meets less frequently, are perhaps more specialized.

In addition to these Performing Arts Medicine journals, journals of other disciplines may also provide an outlet. Examples are the Psychology journals, the Sports Medicine journals and even the journals of Rheumatology and Orthopaedic surgery. The journal Clinical Rheumatology recently devoted the whole of a themed issue to Performing Arts Medicine where a small part of the content of this book also appeared.

If those exemplify the dissemination of information to practitioners and therapists, teachers and performers will be more familiar with a different group of publications. In the UK the Foundations for Excellence series, which emanated from a Dartington conference in 2009 is highly respected and concentrates on educating the music and dance teachers who educate children and adolescent

Musical Impact

Conferences and networking lead to collaboration and research grant applications. Perhaps one of the most successful recent examples of this in the UK, closely related to the UCL MSc degree is the award of a large grant from the Arts and Humanities Research Council for the research project "Musical Impact". Masterminded by Aaron Williamon from the Royal College of Music, this project unites eight of the most important music conservatoires in the UK in a large study on the effects of music making on musicians' health and wellbeing. A cohort of students across the UK, mainly those studying at these elite conservatoires, will be monitored throughout their training for health, injury, psychology and prowess in performance and interactions between these factors will be determined.

In parallel, additional funding will be directed towards Trinity-Laban Conservatoire of Music and Dance for more detailed analysis of the physical and mental demands of practice and performance and to the Royal Northern College of Music for the study of health promotion both in music education and in the profession.

The Future

Performing Arts Medicine is an infant amongst medical specialities. With the exception of sports medicine, it is the only branch of medicine based upon an occupation rather than an organ, a set of diseases or a particular function of the body. It is perhaps therefore fitting that it shares a certain amount with sports medicine, although rationally it might have more in common with occupational medicine.

It differs from sports medicine, which in comparison is awash with money, be it from sponsorship, large crowds of enthusiasts or, in the UK, from the National Lottery. By contrast, financial support tends to be less for the Arts so performers do not have easy access to unlimited medical facilities.

It shares aspects of Occupational medicine, such as hearing damage, but differs in that an artistic element is added to the usually repetitive demands of the workplace even though the principles of musculo-skeletal function are the same in both arenas.

Against this background the surprise is that it has advanced as far as it has since its inception some thirty odd years ago. Perhaps this reflects the dedication of the practitioners and therapists, often from a performing background themselves, together with the challenges of patient care in this specialist and highly complex area. Musicians and dancers are clearly athletes but this athleticism is used in the context of artistic convention as well as artistic interpretation with all the intellectual challenge that implies. This is not always fully understood by wealthy sports doctors.

Whilst this dedication exists, even with the perverse satisfaction of dealing with such complex patients, the future of the speciality is likely to be set fair. Many dancers, on their relatively early retirement, consider a second career in osteopathy or physiotherapy. Some proceed to Dance Science, especially those who, sadly, consider their dance career may have been shortened by access to the best medical attention or, even worse, because of inappropriate medical advice, however well intentioned. The advent of Music Science, partially based on Dance Science, as the newest discipline, will hopefully increase interest in courses such as the UCL MSc which accepts a good degree in one of these two subjects as a qualification for entry. Many of the teachers on that course consider they learn as much from the students as they are able to teach them.

This trend is likely to enhance the network of therapists, dually qualified not just in therapy but also in their own art form. This as well as networking between performers and medics will lead to themed clinics in Performing Arts Medicine, devoted to particular instruments or groups of similar instruments and to particular styles of dance in which knowledge of the particular techniques required combines with medical knowledge to cure a problem and, most important, to prevent it from recurring.

This care will be additionally informed by the results of research projects like "Musical Impact" described above, especially where there is the opportunity to disseminate findings both to the clinicians and to the performers and their teachers.

Ultimately, performing might become almost injury free. At present there is still some way to go.

Bibliography

Books Mainly for Performers

Playing (Less) Hurt: An Injury Prevention Guide for Musicians. Janet Horvath. Self published by Janet Horvath.

An excellent readable guide from a cellist who had to give up her career because of injury.

The Musician's Way: A Guide to Practice, Performance and Wellness. Gerald Klickstein. Published by Oxford University Press, Oxford and New York.

A musicians viewpoint, concentrating an artistry as much as technique.

The Musician's Body: A Maintenance Manual for Peak Performance. Jaume Rosset I Llobet and George Odam. Published by Guildhall School of Music and Drama and Ashgate Publishing Limited.

Simple didactic advice, lavishly illustrated often in cartoon style.

Books on Dance Medicine

Dance Technique and Injury Prevention. Justin Howse. Published by A and C Black, London.

The accepted international textbook on dance medicine written by the orthopedic surgeon to the Royal Ballet with a contribution from Moira McCormack, physiotherapist to the Royal Ballet.

Conditioning for Dance. Eric Franklin. Published by Human Kinetics, Champaign, Illinois.

Good anatomical and physiological analysis of conditioning programmes to assist with safety of dancers.

H.A. Bird, *Performing Arts Medicine in Clinical Practice*,
DOI 10.1007/978-3-319-12427-8,

Books on Instrumental Medicine

Medical Problems of the Instrumentalist Musician. Edited by Raoul Tubiana and Peter Camadio. Published by Martin Dunitz, London.

The accepted international multi-author textbook dealing with all aspects of instrumental medicine.

The Musician's Hand: A Clinical Guide. Ian Winspur and Christopher B Wynn Parry. Martin Dunitz, London.

An excellent multi-author review of hand problems in instrumentalists, compiled by a hand surgeon and a rehabilitationist.

Books on Voice and Voice Medicine

Care of the Professional Voice. D Garfield Davies and Anthony F Jahn. Published by A and C Black, London.

An excellent brief textbook by two clinical otolaryngologists. Could be read in conjunction with Chapter 4.

Voice. Edited by Sir Keith Falkner. Yehudi Menuhin Music Guides. Published by Kahn and Averill, London

The singer's perspective from a UK viewpoint.

On the Art of Singing. Richard Miller. Published by Oxford University Press, New York and Oxford.

The singer's perspective from a USA viewpoint.

Books for the Scientifically Inclined

Musical Excellence: Strategies and techniques to enhance performance. Aaron Williamon. Oxford University Press. Oxford and New York.

An excellent multi-author scientific review of ways in which performance can be enhanced, mainly psychological and physiological aspects.

The Biology of Musical Performance and Performance Related Injury. Alan H D Watson. The Scarecrow Press. Lanham, Maryland, Toronto and Plymouth UK.

An excellent single author book, especially strong on anatomy and neuro-anatomy.

Hypermobility of Joints. Peter Beighton, Rodney Grahame and Howard Bird. Springer. London, Heidelberg and New York.
A comprehensive review of all aspects of joint flexibility with a chapter on Flexibility in the Performing Arts.
The Psychology of Music Performance Anxiety. Dianna T Kenny. Published by Oxford University Press, Oxford and New York.
The sophisticated science of psychological issues in performers.

Index

H.A. Bird, *Performing Arts Medicine in Clinical Practice*,
DOI 10.1007/978-3-319-12427-8,

C

D

MIX
Papier aus verantwortungsvollen Quellen
Paper from responsible sources
FSC® C105338

FSC
www.fsc.org

If you have any concerns about our products,
you can contact us on
ProductSafety@springernature.com

In case Publisher is established outside the EU,
the EU authorized representative is:
Springer Nature Customer Service Center GmbH
Europaplatz 3, 69115 Heidelberg, Germany

Printed by Libri Plureos GmbH
in Hamburg, Germany